Sacred Sanskrit Words

संस्कृत

Sacred Sanskrit Words

for Yoga, Chant, and Meditation

Leza Lowitz and Reema Datta

संस्कृत

Stone Bridge Press • Berkeley, California

Published by
Stone Bridge Press
P.O. Box 8208
Berkeley, CA 94707
TEL 510-524-8732 • sbp@stonebridge.com • www.stonebridge.com

Title page: The word "Sanskrit" (Saṃskṛt) in Devanāgarī script.

The publisher wishes to gratefully acknowledge the developers of Adobe InDesign and of the fonts Sanskrit 99 and Gentium, whose work greatly facilitated the production of this book.

Front-cover design by Michael Rowley.

Printed in the United States of America.

2009 2008 2007 2006 2005 10 9 8 7 6 5 4 3 2 1

ISBN 1-880656-87-6

CONTENTS

INTRODUCTION

A Brief History of Sanskrit

The Sanskrit language was introduced into the highly evolved and urbanized Indus Valley civilization with the Aryan migration of 2500–1500 B.C.E. The Aryans, who were mostly Sanskrit-speaking, tall, fair-skinned, nomadic warriors, migrated to Northwest India from Central Asia (present-day Iran and southern Russia). The fusion of the Aryans with the well-developed native Dravidian culture gave rise to the rich Hindu tradition.

The earliest form of recorded Sanskrit is the *Rig Veda*, which dates back to about 1500 B.C.E. Vedic culture flourished from 1500–500 B.C.E.; the insights and wisdom revealed in the text provided not only the foundation of Hinduism and yoga philosophy but a legacy of literary skill.

As the culture in North India evolved, the Sanskrit language underwent changes. When the language began to diverge from that of the sacred texts, priests and holy men of the Brahmin class became concerned that the hymns might not be preserved and transmitted without corruption. Consequently, they pursued studies of Sanskrit as a language, especially its phonetics. It was the work of the Indian grammarians, in fact, codifying and cataloguing Sanskrit's rules of usage, that led to the development of the field of linguistics. Around 500–350 B.C.E., one of these grammarians, Pāṇini, composed a text on Sanskrit grammar, the *Ashtadhyayi* ("Eight Chapter Grammar"), marking a shift from Vedic to Classical Sanskrit.

Sanskrit houses an enormous pantheon of Hindu gods as reflected in its script, whose name, "Devanāgarī," literally means "language of the gods." Though Sanskrit is written in many scripts, including Telegu, Bengali, and Brahmi, Devanāgarī script is the one most commonly used. In fact, many people believe that Divine Light took the form of the several dozen sacred letters of the Sanskrit language, through which the Divine speaks and resonates even today.

The way in which the development of the Sanskrit language reflects the development of the Hindu religious and philosophical tradition gives it one of the richest spiritual histories of any extant language. Unlike most ancient languages, however, Sanskrit is not dead. It is very much alive. Amazingly, the very words holy men used to record sacred texts twenty-five millennia ago in the form of mantra are still used by their spiritual descendents for the same purposes today. Since Sanskrit is not commonly used for every-day communication, it tends to show less change than languages that are put to more practical use.

One of the most significant uses of Sanskrit was for the recitation of ritual texts. Rituals were performed largely to create a meditative atmosphere for looking inward as well as for connecting with the surrounding nature—all leading to an understanding of the self and the cosmic order. Sanskrit was thus used to explore and describe the subtle and complex realms of metaphysics, cosmology, theology, the workings of the mind and soul, forms of thought, and states of consciousness—areas that were of the highest importance to its creators. And to what end? Ultimately, for the discovery of our own divine nature and an understanding of how to live in harmony with the cosmic order for ultimate well-being and liberation. In the East, Sanskrit continues to exert a powerful influence. Though there are now over a hundred languages and scripts in India, including Tamil, Bengali, Gujarat, Urdu, Pali, and others, Sanskrit continues to be used in the pursuit of the spiritual.

Sanskrit has many words for the Divine and

many terms for defining different levels of consciousness. It is this rich spiritual and mental background that draws contemporary students to Sanskrit today, even in the West. We can gain access to this heritage through the same words the masters used, and by so doing we can touch and be touched by the "spirit of the letter" that touched these sages. And while one can't help but be aware of Sanskrit's longevity, along with this awareness comes the knowledge of our own impermanence, a fact that is in itself a source of liberation from the present moment and its concerns. Though the lessons we learn about ourselves might be contemporary, through Sanskrit we have the opportunity to come into the realm of a sacred language that is timeless, immutable, and eternal.

Introduction to the Sanskrit language provides a key to the philosophical teachings of ancient Hindu literature, from which the ever-popular practice of yoga and the holistic science of Āyurveda evolved. Some of the earliest scriptures on yoga—the practice of which was passed down through oral tradition for thousands of years—were written in Sanskrit about 2,000 to 2,500 years ago.

The keen interest that yoga students show in Sanskrit has surprised us since we began teaching yoga in the San Francisco Bay Area a few years ago.

Some students are mesmerized by the beauty of the sound of the Sanskrit language, others by the artistic look of the Devanāgarī scipt, and many by the world of thought that "karma," "dharma," "ahimsa," "Om," and many other Sanskrit words embody. Musicians, health practitioners, scientists, philosophers, historians, and everyday people have all been profoundly moved by this remarkably scientific language, in which lie all the tools to understand the self and nature and ultimately to connect with the Divine or cosmic source that links us all.

The Sanskrit Alphabet: Pronunciation Guide

The charts below indicate where sounds are articulated in the mouth:

- Guttural: throat
- Palatals: middle of the mouth (at the palate)
- Cerebrals: roof of the mouth (with the tongue bent)
- Dentals: teeth
- Labials: lips

Vowels

Vowels can be short or long. Long vowels are pronounced (or held) twice as long as short vowels and are indicated by a macron written over the letter.

VOWELS: SHORT AND LONG

Guttural	अ	a	(like the first "a" in America)
	आ	ā	(like "a" in father)
Palatal	इ	i	(like "i" in it)
	ई	ī	(like "ee" in sheet)
Labial	उ	u	(like "u" in put)
	ऊ	ū	(like "oo" in food)
Cerebral	ऋ	ṛi	(like "ri" in river)
	ॠ	ṛī	(like "ri" in river, held twice as long)
Dental	ऌ	ḷi	(like "lry" in cavalry)
Diphthongs	ए	e	(like "a" in ate)
	ऐ	ai	(like "ai" in aisle)
	ओ	o	(like "o" in snow)
	औ	au	(like "ou" in loud)
Nasal	अं	aṃ	(nasalized "a" followed by the sound *m*)
Aspirate	अः	aḥ	(echoed "a" with light aspiration)

Consonants

The consonants followed by an "h" are aspirated. "C"

is pronounced "ch" as in chase. "J" is pronounced "j" as in jungle. Consonants marked with a dot below are retroflex, pronounced by rolling the tongue back so that the tip is pointing to the back of the palate. There is a subtle difference between "Ś" as in Śakti and "ṣ" as in ṛiṣi. Both are pronounced "sh," the former as in dish, the latter as in harsh, the tongue retroflexed. "S" is like the s in sour. "M" is pronounced by nasalizing the vowel it precedes and following it with the sound "m." "H" is pronounced by making an echo of the vowel preceding it with a slight aspiration.

Gutturals	Ka क	Kha ख	Ga ग	Gha घ	Ṅa ङ
Palatals	Ca च	Cha छ	Ja ज	Jha झ	Ña ञ
Cerebrals	Ta ट	Tha ठ	Da ड	Dha ढ	Ṇa ण
Dentals	Ta त	Tha थ	Da द	Dha ध	Na न
Labials	Pa प	Pha फ	Ba ब	Bha भ	Ma म

SEMI-VOWELS

Palatal	*Cerebral*	*Dental*	*Labial*
Ya य	Ra र	La ल	Va व

SIBILANTS

Palatal	*Cerebral*	*Dental*	*Labial*
Śa श	Ṣa ष	Sa स	Ha ह

Sanskrit is written from left to right. For each word, all the letters making up the word are written first, and then a horizontal line is added on top of the letters last, showing that the letters under the line make up that word. For example, for the word *āsana* (आसन), first the vowel "a" (अ) is written by making the number "3" and then adding a small horizontal line to connect to the vertical line. To show that the vowel "ā" is long, another vertical line is added (आ). For the "s" sound, the number "2" is written, followed by a small horizontal line connected to a vertical line (स); for the "n" sound, we draw a small circle and, from it, a horizontal line that leads to another vertical line (न). After the three letters are written, a horizontal line is added on top, again made from left to right (आसन). Once written, the phonetic nature of the Sanskrit language makes it very easy to read in the Devanāgarī script.

Sacred Sound

Those who become familiar with the language may find that Sanskrit words are powerful in ways that words from other languages are not.

The sound of each one of the Sanskrit letters is actually considered sacred, with its own vibration and deeply resonating tone. Legend has it that these sacred sounds were born from Lord Śiva's drum itself (although, as if to deliberately confuse the issue, some historical theories have it that Sanskrit sounds and language came much before the mythology of Śiva!). In fact, many people come to Sanskrit these days through sound. If you've ever been in a room full of people chanting the sacred sound *Om*, you know what a transcendent and powerful experience it can be to enter the current of this ancient sound and have it resonate within your own being. The different tones mingle and soar, moving in and out of harmony.

The scientific basis for the Sanskrit language is the idea that sound, made up of vibrations, is energy. According to legend, holy men, or *ṛiṣis,* composed mantras (sacred hymns found in Sanskrit texts) by arranging Sanskrit words in such a way that the sounds not only convey meaning but have the potential to calm, purify, and energize the mind as it vibrates in the different chakras (energy centers) of the subtle body.

The rhythmic repetition of sound—a discipline known as Mantra Yoga—is based on the principle that sound has the power to build consciousness and manifest energy to the point where one can awaken *kuṇḍalinī śakti,* dormant energy lying at the base of the spine. Upon awakening *kuṇḍalinī*, one can achieve *samādhi*, or supreme consciousness. Many schools of Hindu thought, particularly Tantra, believe that sonic consciousness ultimately leads to supreme consciousness.

The *Vedas* state that sound is the easiest, most direct way to connect with the Divine. We have seen in our own practice and teaching that once a practitioner connects with the sound and energy of his/her breath, the heightened consciousness makes it possible then to connect with the sound/energy of a mantra, the sound/energy of a room, and the sound/energy of the surrounding people, plants, and spirits. This then leads toward the realization, ultimately, that it is all one energy, one vibration, originating from the one primordial sound *Om*, from which all of existence begins and dissolves. It does seem that sonic consciousness is the most direct way to realize the state of yoga, the ultimate unity in all things. More and more yoga practitioners are enthusiastically taking to Mantra Yoga, expanding and deepening their experience of yoga.

The word "Sanskrit" means "polished," "refined," or "perfectly composed." Its highly refined nature can be appreciated by understanding the scientific pattern of the sounds and the regulated pronunciation. Sanskrit is devised according to where in the mouth the sounds are made, a direct influence on how much energy one uses to create the sound. Ancient Indians have been called pioneers of the science of phonetics due to the highly refined arrangement of the alphabet.

For every sound in the Sanskrit language there is just one letter, and for every letter, just one sound. It is a phonetic language, the structure of which enables one to write all the phonemes accurately, either as separate consonants and vowels, or syllable to syllable. Sanskrit consists of over two dozen consonants and over a dozen vowels, each of which resides in the different chakras. Every word or sound (*śabda*) has energy and power (*śakti*).

As the ancients knew, sound affects consciousness. The mantra *So Hum* is one example of how sound can affect one's state of mind. When the mind quiets, a practitioner of yoga/meditation can hear that the natural sound of the breath is *So Hum*. The sound vibration of the inhalation is *So*, while that of the exhalation is *Hum*. If one focuses on this sound-vibration, every inhalation can become inspiring and every exhalation a release, resulting in a lightness of mind that allows one to move more freely toward the spirit, truth, and higher consciousness.

Sacred sound awakens the life force that is alive within us, sending it through us and out into the world. The sound simply takes over the body, and before long you can't tell where your voice ends and another begins, where your body ends and another begins.

When we chant together without regard to how we "sound," we're cracking open the most frozen of hearts, and it's impossible not to be moved by the vibrations of these primal, unadorned sounds. That power and aliveness moves us instinctively inward, and we move away from our cluttered, noisy minds into our pure, essential, joyful essence. And we're not just chanting in the here and now. Chanting Sanskrit, we go back centuries, dipping into the stream of those who have made similar inquiries, leading to rich discoveries and profound revelations along the way. Chanting is an act of devotion, and an act of uniting with oneself as well as with others. It's a powerful practice of joy and surrender. Much like yoga or meditation, it's a way of liberating the spirit, of becoming free. When we hear the echoes of our own souls in these sounds, it's like hearing a thousand-year-old temple bell ringing in an old Zen temple. What we hear is the deepest silence. And within that silence is the music of the heart that beats within us all.

Our Offering

We started to put together this primer largely in response to yoga students who wanted to learn Sanskrit chants and terms, and as a guidebook in our own study and teaching. Sometimes students would ask, "What does *Om* mean?" Or, if they were studying the *Vedas* or the *Yoga Sūtras*, they might ask, "What is the difference between *puruṣa* and *prakṛti*?" Often, when there were glossaries or dictionaries available, they didn't have both the English pronunciations and the Devanāgarī script together. So we were intrigued when we were having lunch at a Japanese restaurant on Solano Avenue in Berkeley with our publisher, and he suggested that we create this primer as a kind of sister volume to *Designing with Kanji*, a book on the Japanese ideogram. Though we are far from specialists in Sanskrit, we've found that the best way to learn about something is to write about it, so researching and writing about Sanskrit became our own deep learning process as well.

Most Sanskrit words derive from a particular verb-root (*dhātu*) that reveals the origin of the word. The various terms and philosophies Sanskrit words describe contain subtle but very particular distinctions in terms of meaning according to different schools of Hindu or Buddhist thought. Those distinctions are often contradictory, particularly to the layperson. A Jainist understanding of a word might be different from a Buddhist understanding, for example, and such subtle distinctions are beyond the scope of this book. Though it is precise, Sanskrit is a complex and multifaceted language. For example, it is easy to get lost in the many different names for the gods and their many different and sometimes paradoxical characteristics.

We have therefore tried to simplify the definitions while not omitting important information, but space considerations and the nature of this book have dictated that much of the nuance and complexity associated with these words had to be left out. There are also many debates about the translations of certain key terms. When possible, we have offered alternate translations. However, this book is not intended to be a language textbook. Rather, it is more of a window into an ancient language and the precepts for living that this language illuminates. We hope it inspires people to pursue a more in-depth study of this rich language and its living guides—the *Vedas*, the *Upaniṣads*, the *Bhagavad Gītā*, and the *Yoga Sūtras*, among others. We recommend that those looking for an in-depth discussion of Sanskrit language, grammar, and meaning and of Indian philosophy consult the books listed in the Bibliography. *Sacred Sanskrit Words* is offered as a basic compendium and as a celebration of an ancient Eastern language that has become increasingly popular in the West.

The book is organized in alphabetical order, with the Devanāgarī script and English transliteration of each word given on the same page, along with a definition and relevant facts, myths, history, and quotations. Though there were many words we wanted to include, space limited our entries to words of particular interest to students of yoga, Hindu mythology, and philosophy.

As Sanskrit has become popularized in the West, many alternative spellings and pronunciations have arisen to make the words easier to say. For example, the word *ācārya* (yoga master) is often spelled Acharya, and *Śiva* and *Śakti* are often spelled Shiva and Shakti. We have noted alternative spellings in the entries whenever applicable. And while linguists might not agree, we have added an "s" to form plurals of Sanskrit "nouns"—*Vedas* and *Upaniṣads,* for example—to improve sense and readability in a book intended primarily for laypersons. Sanskrit terms that are very well known as English words (such as yoga, karma, and guru) are treated as English (written in roman type, without diacritical marks). Proper names (Kṛiṣṇa, Śiva, etc.) are written in roman type with diacriticals, as are compounds where one word is Sanskrit and the other is treated as English (Haṭha Yoga, Mahāyāna Buddhism). All other Sanskrit terms are written in italic type, with diacriticals.

Sanskrit Here and Now

Although most young people in India do not study Sanskrit, much as Greek and Latin are not widely studied in the West, Sanskrit words and their meanings continue to affect the everyday lives of most Indians in the form of morning prayers, celebrations of birthdays and marriages, and their perspectives on life and death, joy and suffering, poverty and wealth.

Sanskrit is the root of a great number of languages, including those of Europe and South Asia. Buddhist as well as Hindu texts are written in the Sanskrit language. Buddhism had a deep impact on religion and philosophy in China, which imported many Sanskrit words and concepts. These imports eventually made their way to Japan and are now part of the Buddhist tradition there. Though Buddhism and Hinduism have their differences, concepts such as karma, *māyā*, mantra, reincarnation, yoga, and meditation are common to both.

Sanskrit words and concepts started to crop up in the popular culture of the West over three decades ago, with songs like the Beatle's "Jai Guru Dev Om" and Steeley Dan's "Bodhisattva." Band names like Nirvana and Third Eye Blind, and albums like No Doubt's *Secret Samadhi* or Madonna's *Ray of Light* continue to reflect the interest artists have in Eastern traditions. Sanskrit even began a few years ago to hit Madison Avenue, which is a sure sign of becoming mainstream, at least on the surface. Brand or product names like Tantra, Shanti, Om, Prana, and Shakti appeared by the dozens. Then there was a craze for body painting and henna tattooing, and red dots started to pop up on the foreheads of models and rock stars. In the past few years, more and more people, especially devoted *yogīs* and *yoginīs*, have had *Namaste*, *Om*, or *Jīvanmukti* tattooed onto their bodies as a way to remind them or tell others of their spiritual paths. While most of the tattoos are written correctly (yogīs tend to do their research), occasionally a Sanskrit word has been tattooed upside down, sideways, or out of proportion.

This book offers a basic guide to some of the most significant words in the language and provides the proper Devanāgarī script accompaniment.

In the West today, one can find yoga studios and meditation centers where Sanskrit words, *sūtras*, and scriptures have been copied onto walls or stenciled onto fabrics draped over altars or hung in meditation rooms. The use of Sanskrit emphasizes the realm of all the things the Sanskrit language embodies—spiritual inquiry, devotion, offering, prayer, transcendence. Chants can be copied so they can be studied, meditated upon, or followed while sung. Sanskrit words like *smṛiti* ("mindfulness") can be used on cards, papers, jewelry, textiles, meditation cushions, and clothes to set one's intention or to invoke those qualities in one's life, like a sacred stone or amulet.

Namaste

We offer a thousand and eight lotus blossoms of thanks to Matthew Clark, Alan Finger, Scott Gerson, Shogo Oketani, Danny Paradise, Larry Schultz, Jayant Shroff, our intrepid publisher Peter Goodman, Jaime Starling, Barry Harris, our patient and painstaking editor Elizabeth Floyd, and the talented designer Michael Rowley for helping us bring this book into being. We are grateful to have received the guidance of Sanskrit scholars in Varanasi, England, and the United States, who gave of their time and knowledge anonymously. We thank them from the bottom of our hearts, and acknowledge that any mistakes in the text are ours, not theirs. We give a special thanks to our parents and families for their patient and persistent love and support. We also want to give a special thank you to Hideaki Oketani, whose vast library contained rare books of Hindu philosophy and literature, and to Donna Mendelsohn, who sent shiploads of books overseas in care packages (and thanks also to the American and Japanese postal services for delivering them). *Namaste* also to Windi Braden, our loving and wise spiritual guide. We humbly honor our teachers—past, present, and future—and our students, and all the *bodhisattvas* out there (you know who you are) for giving of yourselves so generously. Thank you!

As we put the finishing touches on this book, a new year has arrived. Each culture around the world acknowledges and celebrates the new year with its own gestures, symbols, and rituals to the Gods. In Japan, people are cleaning their homes to welcome the *toshigami* (the gods of the incoming year) and decorating their doorways with sprigs of pine attached to cut bamboo. They leave rice cakes, tangerines, kelp, and dried persimmon at the family altar as an offering to the spirits.

In India, business owners remove accounting books from their shelves to conduct *pūjā* (prayers) over their pages, bowing to Goddess Lakṣmi, thanking her for the profits of the year past, and requesting blessings for the year to come. Homes vibrate with the serene sounds of Sanskrit prayers, the sweet aroma of homemade milky deserts, and the rich colors of new clothes and decorations. People gather all over the country in homes, temples, and *āśrams* to chant God's many names for hours before the new year strikes. They use their voices and the sounds and vibrations of the Sanskrit language to welcome the new year with bliss, love, and unity. Like them, we know that Sanskrit is a language of offerings. So we make this offering to you, with blessings for peace and happiness, joy and love.

—Om Śānti—

Leza Lowitz
Tokyo, Japan

Reema Datta
Varanasi, India, and on the road

Sacred Sanskrit Words

संस्कृत

अभ्यास
Abhyāsa

"Constant practice," "continuous effort," "repeated endeavor or exertion," "discipline." Originating from the roots *as* ("to throw") and *abhi* ("toward"), *abhyāsa* means "to throw oneself into an endeavor toward a particular aim"—in other words, "to pursue the practice of yoga as a means of achieving spiritual wholeness." According to Mīmāṃsa, which is one of the six orthodox schools of Indian philosophy, *abhyāsa* is one of the six markers (*sad-liṅga*) on the traditional path to understanding the *Vedas*, India's oldest and most sacred scriptures: this understanding ultimately leads to spiritual development and liberation. See also SAD-LIṄGA, VEDA.

आचार्य
Ācārya

A spiritual guide, master, or teacher who passes

down the wisdom of the *Vedas*. From the verb root *car* ("to go") and the prepositional prefix *ā* ("toward"), the term literally denotes a teacher moving a student forward on the path toward enlightenment. The title of *ācārya* is often given by a guru to a learned *yogin* or other teacher under his tutelage, upon the student's mastery of an art. The *ācārya*'s duties include initiating, guiding, and instructing others on the spiritual path. *Ācāra* also refers to behavior, traditions, and established rules of conduct, so an *ācārya* is "someone who knows, and whose life exemplifies, the 'rules' of conduct according to classical principles of yoga." The word is sometimes spelled Acharya in English, and the title Yoga Acharya is used to denote a yoga master. See also VEDA, YOGIN.

अद्वैत
Advaita

From the roots *a* ("not") and *dvaita* ("two"), *advaita* literally means "not two," or "oneness with all." *Advaita* is the term used to express the Indian philosophical and spiritual concept of Nondualism, or the belief that there is only One Reality (*brahman*). Nondualism holds that we are not separate from the Divine, nature, or one another, and that all is one interconnected transcendent reality. *Advaita* is also used to refer to Advaita Vedānta, the first school of Indian philosophy to promote the concept of Nondualism; this school teaches that the individual soul (*jīva*) is not distinct from the Absolute, the Supreme Being (*brahman*). See also BRAHMAN, JĪVANMUKTA.

अग्नि
Agni

The powerful Fire God, one of the main deities celebrated in the *Vedas*. Some see Agni as a symbol of divine will, or the sacred spark of the immortal within each mortal being. While Agni is an internal fire, Agni is also a purifying fire—the heat, light, and energy that burns through illusion and leads a seeker to self-knowledge, ultimate Truth, and a state of bliss. As the Fire God, Agni carries the food offered by the *ṛiṣis* to the Gods from earth to heaven during sacrificial rites; he is sometimes represented as a ram. The square fire pits used by the Vedic Brahmans in these ceremonies were called *agni hotra*. "Thou (Agni) dost create food of all kinds and digest it (after it is taken in): and thus Thou preservest all people like a mother, goading them on towards a better and richer life, towards clearer and broader vision, playing various roles, Thou preservest us all in every way" (from Mandala V, the *Rig Veda,* Gopalacharya). See also Ṛṣi, Śānti.

अमिताभ
Amitābha

From *amita* ("unmeasured") and *ābhā* ("splendor"), "Amitābha" means the "Buddha of Unparalleled Splendor" or the "Buddha of Immeasurable Glory." Amitābha is considered the Buddha of Three Forms: the Absolute and Unconditioned, the Savior of Sentient Beings, and the historical Buddha who came to earth to share his teachings. Dogen said, "The Buddha meditated for six years, Bodhidharma for nine. The practice of meditation is not a method for attainment of enlightenment, it is enlightenment itself." See also Buddha.

अमृत
Amṛita

From the root *mṛita* ("to die," "death") and the prefix *a* ("not"), *amṛita* means that which is undying or immortal. It is used as one of the Goddess Lakṣmi's 108 names, often rendered in English as "the Immortal One" or "the One Who Does Not Die." *Amṛita-rasa* also refers to the nectar of the Gods—a sacred ambrosia that emanates from the crown chakra. In yoga practice, inverted postures like the headstand, or the *viparita karani mudrā* ("inverse-action seal"), are believed to seal in the *amṛita* and prevent this precious energy from leaking out from the crown of the head. In Tantric philosophy, the life-sustaining sexual fluids are considered a form of *amṛita-rasa*—a powerful nectar of immortality. See also Chakra, Rasa, Tantra.

आनन्द
Ānanda

A beloved disciple of the Buddha whose name comes from the root verb *nand* ("to rejoice"), Ānanda reportedly became an *arhat* (a Buddhist saint who has been freed from the cycle of birth and death) on the same day that the first Buddhist council (Sanskrit, *sanghiti*) occurred in Rājagriha (in 499 B.C.E.), to collect and preserve Buddha's teachings after his passing. In this exchange in the Buddhist text *Samyutta Nikaya*, he learns what constitutes a holy life. "The venerable Ānanda said to the Lord, 'Half of this holy life, Lord, is good and noble friends, companionship with the good, association with the good.' The Lord replied: 'Do not say that, Ānanda. . . . It is the whole of this holy life, this friendship, companionship and association with the good.'" When Ānanda reached Arhatship, his seat "shone like the lotus flower touched into bloom by the rays of the sun." Ānanda also means "absolute bliss," "complete joy," and "delight."

अनन्त
Ananta

From *an* ("without") and *anta* ("limit"), Ananta is the Divine Serpent upon whom Lord Viṣṇu reclines. It means "he who is infinite," "he who is not confined by time, space, or the material plane." The masculine form, Ananta, is also one of the fourteen names of Lord Viṣṇu. The Feminine form, Anantā (with a long final "a"), is another name for Pārvatī, Śiva's consort. See also Pārvatī, Śiva, Viṣṇu.

अपान
Apāna

From the roots *an* ("to breathe") and *apa* ("away"), *apāna* literally means "carried-downward breath." It refers to the exhalation, the "dying breath" taken when we literally "expire" as we release the breath. *Apāna* is a downward-moving energy that moves from the pelvic bowl and radiates down, coming to rest in earth energy. It is an open, receptive, vast energy, sometimes called "feminine energy." Its opposite is *prāṇa*, the inhalation, the active breath/energy that rises from the diaphragm. When we direct *apāna* energy upward to meet with pranic energy through the use of the "energy lock" (*bandha*) called *mūla bandha*, we can attain higher states of consciousness and awareness. See also Aṣṭāṅga Yoga (Prāṇāyāma), Bandha, Prāṇa.

आसन
Āsana

From the root *ās* (meaning "to sit" and also "to be"), *āsana* literally means "to sit and be." The cognate term *āsandī* means "stool," suggesting the seat where a Vedic ascetic would sit to meditate or to contemplate the universe. In ancient times and in early sacred texts, *āsana* referred to the platform used to sit on during meditation. Later, in the *Yoga Sūtras* (written by Patañjali in about c.e. 200), the meaning became "physical posture" or "yoga posture." The earliest *āsana*, or yoga postures, were *Padmāsana* (Lotus),

Siddhāsana (Adept's pose), and *Vīrāsana* (Hero's pose). *Āsana*, or "Posture," is the third limb, or stage (*aṅga*), in the Eight Limbs of Yoga (Aṣṭāṅga Yoga) codified in the *Yoga Sūtras*. Thus, *āsana* "seats" the body in a particular posture—standing, sitting, lying down, twisting, inverting, bending backward or forward—leading to physical opening (greater flexibility and improved flow of energy), purification, and spiritual awakening.

The practice of *āsana* (assuming yoga postures) is considered an external spiritual practice, or *bāhira sādhana*, initially to be undertaken under the guidance of a guru, master, or teacher, but eventually to be practiced alone as a meditative discipline where the practitioner is fully connected with the inner teacher. Traditionally, there are thought to be 840,000 yoga *āsanas*, most of which represent the natural postures of animals as well as objects in nature such as mountains, trees, and the sun. Most people practice about 50 *āsanas*, with countless variations and modifications, but usually in set sequences (sun salutations, standing postures, seated postures, meditation, and full relaxation). Practice of *āsana* strengthens the muscles, increases flexibility and strength in the spine and joints, and encourages proper alignment while releasing tension and fatigue. It also promotes healthy functioning of the internal organs. *Āsana* also has spiritual benefits—it promotes inner stability and equanimity and fosters the kind of quiet, reflective mind that makes it possible to observe one's own mental and physical habits and patterns and, finally, become free of them. It balances the gross and subtle body. Practicing *āsana* as a series of meditative movements makes it possible to grow beyond the ego-self, to open the heart and shatter the illusion (*māyā*) of separateness that keeps us isolated from others and disconnected from our own true nature.

Chapter Two, verses 46–48 of the *Yoga Sūtras* states (in Miller's translation):

> *Sthira-sukham-āsanam*
> *Prayatna-śaithilya-anata-samāpattibhyām*
> *Tato dvanda-anabhighātāh*
>
> The posture of yoga is steady and easy.
> It is realized by relaxing one's effort and resting like the cosmic serpent on the waters of infinity.
> Then one is unconstrained by opposing dualities.

Through āsana practice we can find the "seat" of the soul and gain liberation (*mokśa*). See also Aṣṭānga Yoga (Prāṇāyāma), Māyā, Sādhana, Yoga.

आश्रम
Āśram

Also *āshram*. A "place where effort is made." A hermitage; an abode of spiritual practice, study, and meditation. Usually the home of a spiritual leader (guru) and his pupils (*chelas*). Also refers to a stage in the life of the seeker, such as *brahmacharya*, or self-control (one of the five *yamas* of Aṣṭāṅga Yoga). See also AṢṬĀṄGA YOGA, GURU, SṚAM.

अष्टाङ्गयोग
Aṣṭāṅga Yoga

Also Ashṭāṅga Yoga. "Eight-limbed Path." This term refers to the eight limbs, or stages (*āṅga)* of classical yoga practice (*sādhana*) that a *yogin* passes through to attain awakening. These stages, which were first codified in the *Yoga Sūtras* of Patañjali more than two thousand years ago, have many similarities to the

Eightfold Path of early Buddhism. The practice of austerities, breath control, meditation, and development of heat for purification actually share similarities with indigenous spiritual traditions throughout the world, such as those in the Americas, the Middle East, Africa, and the Pacific Islands. This Eight-limbed Path is said to be the route to the removal of afflictions, leading to liberation (*mokśa*).

While the first five limbs are *bāhira sādhana* (external practices), the last three are *saṃyama* (internal practices, also referred to as the three stages of meditation) that can only be undertaken on one's own. Some scholars believe that Patañjali did not write the section of the *Yoga Sūtras* outlining the Eight-limbed Path, but that instead it was later added to his original text. Regardless of its origins, the Eight Limbs of classical yoga are studied and practiced by yoga students around the world today.

The Eight Limbs of Classical Yoga

1. Yama यम

Restraints, or moral discipline. The *yamas* consist of five elements of outward spiritual practice performed to avoid unrighteous behavior:

APARIGRAHA अपरिग्रह

Nonacquisitiveness. In contemporary terms, this could mean to avoid greed and the acquisition of material goods, to avoid grasping for power, and to simplify your life. Be content with what you have. Do not hoard. Share and share alike.

ASTEYA असतेय

Nonstealing. Do not take that which does not belong to you in a material, physical, spiritual, intellectual, or emotional sense. Respect others' boundaries and property.

AHIṂSĀ अहिंसा

Nonviolence. Do no harm. Practice nonviolent words and deeds toward yourself and others. Live peacefully in word, deed, and thought.

BRAHMACHARYA ब्रह्मचर्य

Moderation, self-control, strength of will, sexual restraint. Though this *yama* was originally intended to mean abstinence from sexual activity or depravity for spiritual and religious purposes, it has far-reaching significance today. Even if you do not take a vow of celibacy, be virtuous and loving in thought and action. Do not fall prey to lust, selfishness, over-indulgence, or ego trips. In other words: If you talk the talk, you must walk the walk. You cannot live one way on the yoga mat and another off it. Beware of gurus and teachers who live this kind of double-life.

SATYA सत्य

Truthfulness, sincerity, integrity, honesty, the power of the word. Speak the truth. Tell no lies. Be honest to yourself and others, and the world will reflect that honesty back to you, providing you with all the support you need. See also SATYA.

2. *Niyama* नियम

Observances; self-restraint. The *niyamas* consist of five inner practices to follow in maintaining correct moral principles. These are:

SAṂTOṢA संतोष

Contentment, equanimity, happiness, satisfaction. Practice happiness and contentment, honoring all that you are and all that you have right now in this moment. Know that it is truly enough. Be satisfied with your life on a deep level in the present moment. Enjoy the now.

TAPAS तपस्

Burning zeal, desire to achieve self-realization, purification. Practice discipline and cultivate a fiery spirit. Burn through the ego. Practice endurance, building strength, stamina, and wisdom. Understand that discipline is a form of self-care, not self-deprivation.

SAUCHA शौच

Purity of body and mind. Embrace purity in your body, environment, relationships, communications, and actions. Keep yourself and your life clear and clean, within and without. Care for your soul and the environment.

SVĀDHYĀYA स्वाध्याय
Self-observation, self-study. Be rigorous in looking at yourself. Practice introspection. Study the ancient texts and scriptures, read philosophy to enrich your mind and recite poetry to lighten your heart. Know yourself deeply and authentically, so that you may fully know others. Assess your thoughts and actions. Change what you don't like, relinquish what does not serve you or others well. Embrace what does.

ĪSHVARA PRAṆIDHANA ईश्वरप्रणिधान
Surrender to God or the Divine. Be devoted. Let go of your small self and your ego, throw away willfulness and competition. Embrace a higher source, and trust in its benevolence. Accept the mystery and miracle of life, approach it with a sense of gratitude, awe and wonder.

3. *Āsana* आसन

Yoga postures. An external spiritual practice that helps us attain stillness in mind and body. These powerful poses create strength, flexibililty, vitality and self-awareness, cleansing the body and mind and guiding us to a sense of stillness and unity within and without. See also Āsana.

4. *Prāṇāyāma* प्राणायाम

Breath control; achieving a balanced state of mind

through the steadiness of the breath. *Prāṇāyāma* refers to an array of invigorating and relaxing yogic breathing exercises that help us calm the mind and steady the thoughts, awakening inner peace and cleansing the system.

5. Pratyāhāra प्रत्याहार

Withdrawal of the senses, turning the senses inward, controlling the mind through the control of the senses. Practicing detachment from the vicissitudes of life. Moving beyond the ups and downs of external reality into a greater sense of stillness, ease, and spaciousness, by turning awareness inward.

6. Dhāraṇa धारण

Concentration, fixing the attention on one focal point to gain unbroken contemplation. Fostering equilibrium, equanimity, poise, and grace.

7. Dhyāna ध्यान

Meditation, sitting in stillness as the threshold to union with the Divine. Quieting the mind and opening the heart to allow the radiance of the Divine to nurture, heal, inspire, and enliven.

8. Samādhi समाधि

Super-consciousness, pure contentment, equilibrium, enlightenment, ecstasy (standing outside the ordinary self), enstasy (standing inside the self), bliss, peace, union with the Divine. In this state, the spiritual seeker (*sādak*) loses the individual self and merges with the Universal Spirit. *Samādhi* is the state in which one feels, knows, and revels in the direct presence of the Divine with the entire body and soul. See also SAMĀDHI.

In modern times, Aṣṭāṅga often refers to a branch of yoga reportedly reconstructed from the *Yoga Korunta*, a thousand-year-old manuscript of verses on Haṭha Yoga written on palm leaves and discovered in the 1930s by yoga master Śrī Tirumalai Krishnamacharya and his then-student Śrī Pattabhi Jois, who translated it. Also called Aṣṭāṅga Vinyasa Yoga to differentiate it from Patañjali's Aṣṭāṅga Yoga, it synchronizes *āsana* (yoga postures), *prāṇāyāma* (yogic breathing), and the practice of *mūla*, *uḍḍīyāna*, and *jālaṃdhara bandhas* (forms of internal energy locks) to produce a purifying internal heat. See also AṢṬĀNGA YOGA (PRĀṆĀYĀMA), PATAÑJALI, SAMĀDHI, YOGA SŪTRA.

आत्मन
Ātman

Also *ātma* आत्म. Thought to derive from either the root *at* ("to breathe") or the root "*ap*" ("to pervade," "to reach up to"), *ātman* is the transcendental self—one's true nature, or the highest form of self—as distinct from the level of the ego, individuality, or personality. According to the *Upaniṣads*, *ātman* is the ultimate existence of the universe and the vital breath of human beings.

आयुर्वेद
Āyurveda

From *āyur* ("life knowledge," "life science," or "the science of daily living") and *veda* ("to know"), Āyurveda is sometimes called "the knowledge of longevity." This five-thousand-year-old traditional Indian medical science was created from the directly realized knowledge and subsequent practical experience of *ṛiṣis* in ancient India, then passed down through oral tradition and eventually recorded in the *Vedas.*

At the core of Ayurvedic science is the concept that the five elements of nature (earth, water, fire, air, and ether) present themselves as elements in the body. In Ayurvedic science, the body is made up of *dhātus* (tissue), *malas* (waste products), *srotas* (channels), and *doṣas* (energetic forces), which the *Tridoṣas*—or three body types: *kapha* (Earth/Water); *pitta* (Fire/Water); and *vāta* (Air/Ether)—help to create, regulate, and maintain.

Vāta regulates body movement, elimination, metabolism, heart functioning, musculature, and sense perception. *Pitta* also regulates metabolism, as well as body temperature, vision, comprehension, and appetite. *Kapha* regulates structure, lubrication, stability, fertility, and strength. *Vāta* is considered the most important of the three, because an imbalance in *Vāta* can cause the other two *doṣas* to become imbalanced. Āyurveda posits that we all contain unique proportions of the *doṣas*, each of which serve particular functions in the body. However, one *doṣa* is usually dominant in our constitution. Mental, physical, and spiritual health and balance can only be achieved when the individual is in harmony both with nature and with his or her own fundamental nature.

Each *doṣa* has specific characteristics and needs that can be balanced or weakened by diet, environment and lifestyle. *Kapha* is considered the most grounded *doṣa*, embodying stability, patience, and openness. People with this constitution usually have a large build, high body weight, and calm mental activity. When this *doṣa* is imbalanced, one can become lethargic and feel "weighted" to the earth. *Pitta* types are medium in build and weight. Those with a dominant *pitta doṣa* are often fiery, passionate, active types. *Pitta* imbalance can lead to irritation, aggression, and anger. *Vata* types are small, thin, and restless. This *doṣa* has the quality of dryness, coldness, and mobility. *Vata* individuals are more ethereal, creative, and spontaneous types. When imbalanced, those in whom this *doṣa* is dominant can be noncomittal, unreliable, or flighty.

Modern life and all its stresses can impair the body's natural functioning. Ayurvedic healing restores it by keeping the *doṣas* in balance through specific types of exercise, environmental modifications (temperatures, seasons), food, daily activities, colors, sounds, and cleansing procedures best suited to each of these constitutions.

बन्ध
Bandha

From the verb root *bandh* ("to bind"), *bandha* means "lock," "bind," "bond," bondage." In Indian philosophy, bondage is traditionally considered the result of ignorance (*avidyā*) or of karma. The bonds of ignorance can be broken through study and wisdom (*jñāna*). In yogic breathing, or *prāṇāyāma*, there are also three major *bandhas*, or "energy locks," used to help seal in the life force energy (*prāṇa*) during yoga practice, meditation, or *mudrās*. They are:

Jālaṃdhara bandha जालंधरबन्ध
Jāla means "net," "web," or "mesh." An energy lock in which the chin is lowered toward the chest, which rises to meet it. Used during *prāṇāyāma*, or yogic breathing practice. Cleans nasal passages, regulates bloodflow to heart, head, and endocrine glands in the neck (thyroid, parathyroid).

Uḍḍīyāna bandha उड्डीयानबन्ध
Uḍḍīyāna means "flying up." Energy lock in which the abdominal muscles are pulled in and up toward the spine. Engaging this internal lock strengthens the

solar plexus, expands lung capacity, and helps keep the spine erect and the digestive system toned and strong.

Mūla bandha मूलबन्ध

Mūla means "root," origin," or "source." Energy lock in which the anus and perineum (and, in women, the Kegel muscles as well) are lifted. Many yoga practitioners consider *mūla bandha* to be the secret to maintaining strong life-force energy. *Mūla bandha* is a grounding, centering force that helps to create heat, protects the overstretching of muscles, and increases the functioning of the parasympathetic nervous system that is responsible for relaxation. Engaging *mūla bandha* thus creates a relaxed state in the midst of deep movement.

Another important energy lock is *Śiva bandha*, in which the tongue is placed on the upper palate, where the teeth meet the gums, to deepen the effects of *prāṇāyāma*, or yogic breathing. See also APĀNA, AṢṬĀṄGA YOGA (PRĀṆĀYĀMA), PRĀṆA.

भगवद्गीता
Bhagavad Gītā

From the roots *bhaj* ("to love") and *ga* ("to sing") and usually translated as "Song of the Beloved" or "Song of the Lord." This phrase is the title of a 700-verse scripture contained within the 100,000-verse *Mahābhārata* (in Book VI, Chapters 13–40). The *Bhagavad Gītā* is considered one of the essential Hindu scriptures. It was written between the fifth century B.C.E. and the second century C.E. and is attributed to the sage Vyasa. It is one of the oldest known texts on yoga, which itself dates back more than 3,500 years. The *Gītā*, as it is commonly called in modern times, tells the story of two warring clans, the Kauravas and the Pāṇḍavas. The warrior Prince Arjuna, leader of the Pāṇḍavas, confides to his charioteer (who is really Lord Kṛiṣṇa) his reluctance to order the battle to begin at Kurukshetra, since this will make him responsible for the deaths of his own family members. Lord Kṛiṣṇa explains to Arjuna that as a member of the warrior caste he has a duty to fight. If Arjuna takes decisive action, he will be fulfilling his duty—which is the highest possible action—rather than obeying his ego. Kṛiṣṇa reveals to Arjuna that being alive means actively opposing evil by keeping one's actions beyond the grip of the ego. Kṛiṣṇa patiently explains to Arjuna the Trimārga, or the Threefold Path of Yoga, and helps him to overcome his doubts and fears. The Threefold Path consists of: Bhakti Yoga (the yoga of devotion), Jñāna Yoga (the yoga of wisdom, meditation, and asceticism), and Karma Yoga (acting while renouncing the fruits of the action). Finally, Kṛiṣṇa reveals that it is Karma Yoga that Arjuna must practice. Kṛiṣṇa states, "He who gives up action, falls. He who gives up only the reward, rises." Emboldened, Arjuna takes action and orders the battle to begin. Kṛiṣṇa has taught Arjuna how to maintain goodness in the world, and ultimately to attain Godhood. The *Gītā* also describes four types of *yogī*—the sufferer, the seeker of material goods, the seeker of knowledge, and the man of wisdom. In the Vedantic tradition, the *Bhagavad Gītā* is called *Smṛiti Prasthāna*, or the "Remembered Foundation"; the name reflects both its origins as an oral history and its "recollection" of the wisdom we all possess within and are capable of invoking. See also BHAKTI YOGA, GUṆA, JÑĀNA YOGA, KARMA YOGA, KṚIṢṆA.

भक्ति
Bhakti

From the root *bhaj*, "to love and revere." Bhakti refers to devotion to the Beloved—that is, to God or the Divine. Bhakti Yoga is a path of yoga in which the disciple devotes his practice to God as a spiritual offering.

भक्तियोग
Bhakti Yoga

The yoga of devotion. One of the triumvirate of classical yoga known as the Trimārga, or the Threefold Path of Yoga, which also includes Karma Yoga and Jñāna Yoga. Bhakti Yoga is the path to self-realization and union with the ultimate force of the universe (*brahman*), in which a practitioner cultivates faith and devotion, surrendering to the Divine. This is achieved by channeling one's energy and devotion through postures, chanting, singing, scriptural study, ritual, and service to one's particular divinity. Sanskrit is central to this path, as it is the language of the sacred scriptures, chants, and mantras used for devotional practice. The practice of *kirtan*, or devotional chanting, is a central practice of Bhakti Yoga, when one sings wholeheartedly in praise of the gods.

Bhakti Yoga is based on complete faith and surrender to God, but it is not a passive surrender; indeed, one's whole being is active in the process. In India and elsewhere, *sādhus* may spend years in a particular pose, losing all muscle tone and feeling in certain body parts, essentially giving up the physical "envelope" of the body in devotion to the Divine. Or they may spend their entire lives rolling through the streets, naked but for a thin covering of ash, as a form of devotional worship. See also Bhagavad Gītā, Jñāna Yoga, Karma Yoga, Rāja Yoga, Sādhu.

बिन्दु
Bindu

Also *bindi* बिन्दि. "Dot," "seed," or "point"; can also mean "semen." This is a point where the Divine

Energy (*kuṇḍalinī śakti*) converges to create the potential to manifest itself in the universe. In India, you will often see people with a red dot painted between the eyebrows on their forehead at the sixth chakra, the most potent physical point on the body. This dot symbolizes the Third Eye and the inner knowledge and wisdom that connect us to the sacred. This dot is also called *tilaka* or *tika* when made in a ritual offering (*pūjā*) before practice. It is often made from *kum-kum* ("red-red"), which contains a mixture of turmeric, iodine, camphor, and other substances and has a cooling effect. It can also be made of ground sandalwood and musk. *Yogīs* or *sannyāsīs* (monks, ascetics, or spiritual devotees) often use ash for their *tilaka bindi*, as this substance—the result of fire—represents their renunciation of the material plane. The *bindhu* is also found at the center point of *yantra*, a geometrical diagram used in meditation to connect with the Divine that lives in the entire cosmos. See Kuṇḍalinī Śakti, Yantra.

बोधि
Bodhi

Enlightenment; a state of being awakened. Known as *nirvāṇa*, this is the ultimate state of being. The Buddha reached *bodhi* under the Bodhi (fig) tree in India. Buddhist scholar Gary Gach has pointed out the significance of the Bodhi tree as the place of Buddha's enlightenment: fig trees are parthenogenic, rerooting their own branches in the soil, and as such, they are forever self-renewing. See also BUDDHA, NIRVĀṆA.

बोधिसत्त्व
Bodhisattva

"One who is on his way to Buddhahood"; a "Buddha-in-waiting." A *bodhisattva* is a *sattva* (being) who seeks to attain *bodhi* (enlightenment) so that he may be of service to others, spreading the teachings of Buddha and guiding others on the path to liberation. In the

1880s, Lafcadio Hearn described the *bodhisattva* in "The Lotos of Faith":

> In the years when Brahmadatta reigned over Benares—the holy city—the city of apes and peacocks,—the city possessing the seven precious things, and resounding with the ten cries, with the trumpeting of elephants, the neighing of horses, the melody of instruments and voices of singing girls,—then the future Buddha-elect was born as a son in the family of the royal treasurer, after having passed through *kotis* of births innumerable. Now, the duration of one *koti* is ten million years. And the Buddha-elect, the Bodisat, was brought up in splendid luxury as a prince of the holy city, and while yet a boy mastered all branches of human knowledge, and becoming a man succeeded his father as keeper of the treasury. But even while exercising the duties of his office, he gave rich gifts to holy men, and allowed none to excel him in almsgiving.

In Mahāyāna Buddhism, the *bodhisattva* path is not the renunciation or deferral of full Buddhahood until enlightenment is attained by all creatures (as is commonly believed), but rather the commitment to remain in the material plane *as enlightened beings* in order to help all others attain enlightenment. Only when the *bodhisattva*'s mission is accomplished will he leave his physical body and enter the Ultimate Reality. The Four Vows of the Bodhisattva are:

Beings are numberless, I vow to awaken them.
Delusions are inexhaustible: I vow to end them.
Dharma gates are boundless; I vow to enter them.
Buddha's way is unsurpassable: I vow to become it.

ब्रह्मा
Brahmā

"He who has expanded"; the Creator of the Universe. In Hindu tradition, the evolution and the existence of the Universe is the result of the dynamic interplay of three forces, symbolized by the three Gods of the Hindu Trinity, or *Trimūrti.* These are Brahmā (the Creator); Viṣṇu (the Sustainer); and Śiva (the Destroyer). The three cosmic principles they represent—creation, sustenance, and destruction—are present on every level of existence, from the macrocosmic to the microcosmic, from the Universal to the Individual. They are embodied in the cycle of birth, life, death, and rebirth and play out on every level of being, from the physical to the spiritual. Though the three deities are represented individually, they are considered aspects of the same Supreme Force. Yet

they have very distinct characteristics and qualities. Brahmā, the Creator of the Universe, is considered the father of all beings, though he emerged from Viṣṇu's navel in a lotus flower. He is red-skinned and has four heads, from which the four *Vedas* are said to have been born. It is believed that Brahmā created a Goddess (Gāyatrī/Sarasvatī) from within his own body, in order to create the human race. He also has four arms. He holds a cup, a bow (or sometimes a prayer book), a spoon, and the *Vedas*, which he created and disseminated. He is the only one of the *Trimūrti* who does not carry a weapon. Brahmā sits in *Padmāsana* (the Lotus posture), and when he needs transportation he is carried on the back of a white swan. The swan has magical powers, enabling her to separate divine nectar (*soma*) from water and to cull good from evil. Brahmā reigns over *Brahmāloka* (the realm of Brahmā), encompassing the plane of the entire earth and other worlds. He is also believed to control the daily movement of light to dark. The related word *brahman* means Absolute Reality as manifested by Brahmā. A "Brahmin" is "one who knows Brahmā."
See also BRAHMAN, SARASVATĪ, ŚIVA, TRIMŪRTI, VIṢṆU.

ब्रह्मन्
Brahman

From the root *bṛh* ("to expand"). *Brahman* is the Ultimate Reality, the Absolute, the cosmic principle of existence, the Divine, Greater than the Greatest, the Supreme, God. Brahman the Divine is considered infinite and all-pervasive, both physically and metaphysically, and is believed to be the foundation of the universe and the "abode of all consciousness." Everything in the world—mental, spiritual, and material—contains the essence of *brahman*, which is pure existence and pure consciousness. In the *Upaniṣads*, *brahman* is called "*satcidānanda*"—from *sat* ("absolute existence"), *cit* ("absolute consciousness"), and *ānanda* ("absolute bliss"). *Brahman* manifests in each individual as the Supreme Self. Yoga reminds us that there is something larger and more eternal than the "little self"—something beyond the ego or the physical body. When we practice yoga and meditation, we come to realize that we are part of a much larger force that unifies all living things. By looking deeply inside the little self, we "expand" to the bigger Self, the Absolute—or *brahman*—and know that we are part of a larger cosmic whole. See also Ātmaṇ.

ब्राह्मण
Brāhmana

One endowed with purity and wisdom, who has understood *brahman* (the Ultimate Reality) and who spreads the wisdom of the *Vedas*. *Brāhmaṇas* are the liturgical texts used to describe the rituals and rites of the *Saṃhitās,* collections of ancient Vedic hymns.

ब्रह्मविहार
Brahmā-Vihāras

"Dwelling in Absolute Reality." According to Buddhism, there are four sublime states or characteristics of a bodhisattva, or one who has attained liberation. These states are the four *Brahmā-Vihāras,* namely:

Karuṇā करुणा
Compassion, reflecting the belief that one should feel sympathy for others in pain, be they friends, enemies, or complete strangers.

Maitra मैत्र
Love (sometimes translated into the Pali word *metta*, meaning lovingkindness).

Upekṣa उपेक्ष
Equanimity.

Mudita मुदित
Joy; sympathetic joy. An overwhelming sense of joy in life and all that is.

बुद्ध
Buddha

"Awakened One." Someone who has attained enlightenment, or *bodhi*. Though there are many enlightened beings in many different traditions, it is Gautama ("best on earth") or Siddhārtha ("attained goal") to whom we generally refer to when we speak of "the

Buddha." Born in 624 B.C.E. in the foothills of the Himalayas in current-day Nepal, Siddhārtha enjoyed a life of privilege as a prince in the Śakya clan, son of Queen Mayadevi and King Śuddhodana. He is also called Śakyamuni Buddha, from Śakya (his clan name) and *muni* ("able one"). Though his father sheltered him and gave him numerous palaces and material riches, on four occasions he ventured away from the palace and encountered a very different reality. Each time, he came upon a "sign"—an old man, a sick man, a corpse, and a monk. These signs embodied the suffering of humanity and represented Siddhartha's destiny as a spiritual teacher. He renounced his life of leisure, left his wife and son, and traveled east to study Buddhism with various teachers. Eventually he left his teachers and continued wandering on his own, living as an ascetic for nine years. Fearing that his pursuit had been worthless, he sat beneath the Bodhi tree and began to meditate on the Middle Way, the path of nondualism. Forty-nine days later, he attained enlightenment. He gave his first sermon at the Deer Park in Banaras, and devoted the rest of his life to teaching and spreading Buddhism and the possibility of enlightenment. Among his last words, as Gach notes, is this teaching: "Be a lamp unto yourself. Don't look for the answer outside yourself. Hold onto the truth like a torch." See also AMITĀBHA, BODHI, MAHĀYĀNA, MAITREYA.

बुद्धि
Buddhi

From the root *budh* ("to wake up," "know," "understand"). The causative root *bodhaya*, taken from *budh*, can mean "to cause to awaken"; hence, to enlighten. *Buddhi* represents the higher mind, the discriminating mind, higher intelligence, reason, intellectual faculty, and mental perception. The *Katha-Upaniṣad*, which is one of the earliest texts on yoga, written in approximately 1000 B.C.E., promulgates the "yoga of the deep self" (*adhyātma-yoga*), which views the Supreme Being as lying hidden in the deepest recesses of the human heart. In the *Katha-Upaniśad*, the self is described as the charioteer and the body as the chariot. The discriminative faculty (*buddhi*) is the driver, the mind (*manas*) is the reins, and the senses are the horses. When the mind is unyoked from the body, the senses are like wild, uncontrollable horses. But when the mind is yoked, the senses are horses who gently follow along the driver's path, and the self is unified.

चक्र

Chakra

From the root *car* ("to move"), *chakra* can also mean "wheel," "circle," "center," "disc," "sphere." In yogic practice, it refers to wheels of energy. According to yogic and Tantric philosophy, there are seven major chakras or wheels of energy in the human body, and hundreds of minor ones. The body has a central channel of subtle energy, the *suṣumṇa nāḍi*, which runs inside the spine, and two other channels of energy running from the right nostril to the crown of the head and then down the spine (*piṅgalā nāḍi*), and an equivalent channel on the left side (*iḍā nāḍi*). Six chakras are located at the specific points these right and left channels intersect with the central channel. The seventh chakra is located at the crown of the head. Some also believe there is an eighth chakra, the Soul Star, or Transpersonal Chakra, that links the soul/spirit to matter and to its true essence. Each chakra has a particular consciousness. It regulates, distributes, and balances the energy and nerve functions of the area where it is located. It also has an associated color, mantra, tone, sound vibration, image, God or Goddess, sense, *tattva* (element), and *kośa* (layer of experience). The cosmic energy (*kuṇḍalinī śakti*) lies dormant at the base of the spine. When the chakras are activated through yoga, meditation, mantra recitation, or other spiritual practices, the *kuṇḍalinī* energy rises along the central channel, the *suṣumṇa nāḍi*, and activates the chakras, ultimately reaching the crown, the center of higher consciousness and bliss. When the chakras are "whirling" in a bright, balanced, and attuned way, our minds, bodies, and spirits are working in harmony. From top to bottom, the seven chakras are:

Sahasrāra सहस्रार — Seventh Chakra

From the Sanskrit meaning "thousand-fold" or "thousand-petaled." The seventh, or crown, chakra is located at the top of the head. It is considered the center of transcendence, the point from which the spirit leaves the physical body for higher realms. This chakra is associated with spirituality. It symbolizes the higher mind, cosmic intelligence, and union with the Absolute. It governs the central nervous system, upper skull, cerebral cortex, and skin, and revitalizes the cerebrum. Element: none. Associated gland: pineal. Image: A halo or full moon made of a thousand white petals, representing infinity, rapture, bliss, with each petal opened to the highest state of consciousness. Color: white, gold, or violet. Deities: Para-Brahman, Śiva. Mantra: Silence, or the *bija* (seed) mantra *Om*. Tone: B (ti). Vowel sound: ē.

Ājña आज्ञा — Sixth Chakra
From the Sanskrit term meaning "to perceive," "to know." The sixth chakra is the third-eye chakra, located in the brain but depicted between the eyebrows on the forehead. Element: light. Also known as the "guru chakra." Considered the center of inner wisdom, intuition, wisdom, and individuality, this chakra governs the eyes and the base of the skull. Sense: cultivation of the "sixth sense." Associated gland: pituitary. Image: blue-gray two-petaled lotus, with the petals outstretched like wings on each side of a circle that represents two realities. The wings symbolize the ability to transcend the physical realm and enter the spiritual realm. Colors: purple, indigo. Deities: Paramaśiva and Hakini. Mantra: The *bija* (seed) mantra *Om*. Tone: A (la). Vowel sound: i/ē.

Vishuddha विशुद्ध — Fifth Chakra

From the Sanskrit term for "pure" or "purification." The fifth chakra is located at the throat and known as the throat chakra. Element: ether. Considered the center of communication, self-expression, poetry, speaking truth, and inner listening. *Amṛita*, the nectar of immortality, pours forth from this chakra. Governs the functioning of the mouth, lungs, and skin. Sense: sound. Associated gland: thyroid. Image: sixteen-petaled blue lotus, each petal containing a Sanskrit vowel. Inside the lotus is a downward-facing triangle, representing speech; a full moon, and Airavata, a white, many-tusked elephant. Color: blue. Deities: Ardhanarishvara and Shakini. Mantra: *Ham*. Tone: G (so). Vowel sound: ē/eh.

Anāhata अनाहत — Fourth Chakra

From the Sanskrit for "unstruck," referring to the natural sound of the cosmos, a sound that is not made by "striking" an instrument, but instead one that is inherently present in all living things. The fourth chakra is the heart chakra, located at the heart center, the abode of the primordial sound (*śabda*). Element: air. Considered the center of compassion, self-forgiveness, love, and relationships, this chakra governs the functioning of the heart and lungs.

Sense: touch. Associated gland: thymus. Image: blue or green twelve-petaled lotus around a six-pointed star made of two triangles. The downward-facing triangle symbolizes spirit descending into matter (the physical body), the upward-facing triangle, matter rising to join spirit. Color: green. Deities: Isha and the Goddess Kakini. Mantra: *Yam*. Tone: F (fa). Vowel sound: ā/ay.

Maṇipūra मणिपुर — Third Chakra
From the Sanskrit meaning "lustrous gem." Known as the solar plexus chakra, the third chakra is located at the navel. It is considered the center of personal power, will, manifestation. Element: fire. This chakra governs the functioning of the digestive system, the back, spleen, stomach, and abdomen. Sense: sight. Associated gland: pancreas. Image: yellow ten-petaled lotus with a downward-facing triangle within it, surrounded by three *svāstikas*—which are ancient Hindu symbols of Fire (the Fire God, Agni) and self-transformation. Color: yellow. Deities: Lakini and Rudra. Mantra: *Ram*. Tone: E (mi). Vowel sound: aw/ah.

Svādhiṣhṭhāna स्वाधिष्ठान — Second Chakra
From the Sanskrit meaning "sweetness." Also translates as "one's own place," "base," or "support of life."

The second chakra, or sacral chakra, is located at the spleen/genital area. It is considered the center of creativity and sexual energy, survival, and the fulfillment of physical needs. Element: water. This chakra governs the functioning of the reproductive system. Sense: taste. Associated gland: reproductive organs. Image: orange/crimson six-petaled lotus containing a white circle that represents water, and a light blue crescent moon that represents the light visible within the darkness and the yin/yang balance. Inside the moon is a *makara*, an eel-like water creature that symbolizes sexuality and passion. Color: orange. Deities: Viṣṇu and Rakini. Mantra: *Vam*. Tone: D (re). Vowel sound: ō/oh.

Mūlādhāra मूलाधार — First, or Root, Chakra
From the Sanskrit term for "root" or "support." The root chakra. The first chakra is located at the perineum, where the *kuṇḍalinī śakti* is coiled. Element: earth. This chakra is considered the center of physical and material existence, health, survival. Some versions show a snake coiled around a liṅga, representing *kuṇḍalinī śakti* and male sexuality/creative power. Governs the functioning of the legs. Sense: smell. Associated gland: adrenal. Image: red lotus with four petals encompassing a downward-facing triangle

set within a square. Color: yellow. Deity: Gaṇeśa (the Elephant God). Mantra: *Lam.* Tone: middle C. Vowel sound: ū/ooo.

See also AGNI, GAṆEŚA, KUṆḌALINĪ ŚAKTI, LIṄGA, NĀḌI (IḌĀ, PIṄGALĀ, SUṢUMṆA NĀḌI).

चित
Cit

From the verbal root *cit*—"to be aware of, perceive, know." Represents ultraconsciousness, superawareness. It also means "spirit" and "consciousness" and is sometimes written *chit.*

चित्त
Citta

Variously translated as "consciousness," "thought," "mind." There is not one *citta*, but many. *Citta,* or consciousness, is composed of three aspects: *manas*, the lower mind (or the "gathering mind"), that part of the mind that is bound to sense perception; *buddhi*, the higher mind, or intelligence; and *ahaṃkāra*, the ego, or individual identity. This concept appears in the most often-quoted phrase of the *Yoga Sūtras* (Chapter 1, Verse 2), which lays out the foundation of yoga: *Yogaḥcitta vṛitti nirodhah*, which can be translated as "Yoga is that which stills the fluctuations of the mind." Another word, *bodhicitta,* combines *bodhi* (awakening) and *citta* (mind) to mean the "awakened heart" or the "awakened mind." See also Bodhi, Buddhi.

दर्शन

Darśana

Also *darshana*. "Sight," "vision," "philosophical system." Has the dual meaning of "seeing/being seen" and "reflecting," which can refer to self-reflection and mirroring. The term also means "vision of reality." This "vision" can be literal or metaphorical: to physically see or be in the presence of a holy being, Divine Presence, or sacred place; or to perceive reality on a deeper level. *Darśana* is commonly understood to mean "philosophy" or "metaphysical system." In classical Indian philosophy, there are six main *darśanas*: *vaisheshika darśana* (analysis/characterization of the universe; Atomism); *nyaya darśana* (Logicism); *saṃkhya darśana* (philosophical classification of the universe that distinguishes *tattvas* [elements; principles of the universe] from *puruṣa* [the individual soul]); *yoga darśana* (the union of individual consciousness with universal consciousness); *mīmamsa darśana* (ritual interpretation of the *Vedas*; formal religion); *vedānta darśana* (metaphysical inquiry into the self, the universe, and God). These differing but complementary philosophies all share an underlying belief in karma (cycles of birth, death, and reincarnation) and belief in the possibility of transcending one's karma through *mokśa*, or liberation.

देव
Deva

"Higher being," "being of light." From the root *div* ("to shine"). One who radiates or shines; a celestial being.

देवनागरी
Devanāgarī

Deva means "god," and *nāgara* means "city"; *devanāgarī* literally means "divine city." This term for the most commonly used Sanskrit script has its origins in the fact that it was used for holy writings and temple scripts. Some modern Indian languages use variations on this script, and Hindi still uses the original Devanāgarī, with some additions to account for sounds of Persian and Arabic origin.

देवी
Devī

From the root *div* ("to shine"). Shining; radiant Goddess; Śakti. Devī was Lord Śiva's lover, who embodies the energy of the cosmos, or Śakti. This Hindu Goddess is often depicted as the twelve-armed warrior created by Brahmā, Viṣṇu, and Śiva to kill the buffalo-demon Mahishasura, who terrorized the Universe. There are said to be over 33,000,000 different Devis, which are all aspects of the Primordial Goddess. Her benevolent form is known as Pārvatī, while her malevolent form is Kālī Durgā. A prayer to Devi is often chanted in yoga practice:

PRAYER TO DEVI
(Chant each line twice)

Kālī Durga Ānanda Mai
Sarasvatī Devī Ānanda Mai

To warrior and protector goddesses Kālī and Durgā, mothers of bliss

Uma Pārvatī Ānanda Mai
Sarasvatī Devī Ānanda Mai

To Sarasvatī, pure Goddess of wisdom and the arts, mother of bliss

Sarasvatī Devī Ānanda Mai
Kālī Durga Ānanda Mai

To Śiva's Śakti, Umā, and Pārvatī, mothers of bliss

धर्म
Dharma

"Duty," "righteousness," "law and order," "religion." From the verb root *dhr* ("to hold," "to establish," "to support"), *dharma* literally means "that which holds together." In both Buddhist and Jainist traditions, *dharma* is considered to be the underlying moral structure of the universe. Following one's *dharma*, or duty, is the path to liberation. The term can also refer to the teachings of the Buddha, as well as everything to which they pertain. As Tyberg notes, the great modern sage Śrī Aurobindo said, "*Dharma* is both that which we hold to and that which holds together our inner and outer activities, and in this its primary sense, it means a fundamental law of our nature which secretly conditions all our activities, and in this sense each type, species, individual group has its own *dharma*."

दीक्षा
Dīkshā

Initiation. From the roots *da* ("to give") and *ksha* ("to destroy"), *dīkshā* refers to the process by which an adept or disciple is inducted into a lineage or school of traditional yoga, or taught secret rituals or practices, which helps destroy the bonds of ego and lead one toward a state of grace. Scholar Monier Williams has suggested that *dīksh* is an independent verb meaning "to consecrate," which is derived from *daksh*, "to be able" or "to be strong."

दीपावली
Dīpāvalī

"Row of lights." Among the most important of the Hindu holidays, Dīpāvalī marks the New Year on the Hindu calendar and celebrates the triumph of light over darkness, good over evil, knowledge over ignorance, and justice over injustice. Though its significance varies regionally, it is most often celebrated as the day Lord Kṛiṣṇa kills the demon Narakasura; the day Lord Rāma returns to Ayodhyā after defeating his rival, Rāvana; and the day Lakṣmi, Goddess of wealth, marries Lord Viṣṇu. Homes are cleaned and decorated with earthen oil lamps, signifying the power of light to dispel the darkness from within us and from our surroundings. The upward movement of the flame denotes a path toward knowledge and divinity. Children light fireworks, wear new clothes, and decorate the entrance of their homes with colorful "rangoli" patterns symbolizing welcome and revelry. The clean homes and bright lights are said to attract Lakṣmi, who blesses her devotees with wealth and prosperity. Often referred to as the "festival of lights," Dīpāvalī is a day when people pray for illumination and prosperity on both the spiritual and physical planes. Also known as Diwālī or Divālī.

दृष्टि
Driṣṭi

Meaning "gaze," "view," "sight," *driṣṭi* is from the root *dṛsh* ("to see," "perceive," "understand"). The *driṣṭi* is the point of focus, or "looking place," assigned to each *āsana*, or yoga posture. Maintaining a steady gaze is an important part of yoga, as it focuses the senses, harnesses the mind, and allows the *yoginī* to stay centered in her own inner experience rather than gazing outward or focusing on the external. This gaze ultimately leads to *samadriṣṭi*, or "equal vision"—a state of equanimity in which the *yoginī* sees herself as akin to everything in the world, viewing all things as equal and ultimately seeing the Divine in everything. There are nine different *driṣṭi* in yoga practice: *nasagrai* (the tip of the nose); *broomadhya* (the third eye); *nabi chakra* (the navel); *hastagrai* (the hands); *padhayoragrai* (the toes); *pārśva driṣṭi* (to the far left or far right); *angusta ma dyai* (the thumb); and *ūrdhva driṣṭi* (to the sky).

दुःख
Duḥkha

From *dur* ("bad") and *kha* ("state"), this term is commonly used to mean "sorrow," "grief," "impermanence," "suffering," "dissatisfaction," "stress," "craving," "attachment." The original meaning was "bad axle space," referring to a chariot wheel that was improperly aligned, leading to a bumpy ride and difficulty negotiating turns. *Duḥkha* refers to the human condition, which is one of suffering, as long as we remain in ignorance (*avidyā*) of *ātman*, our true transcendent nature. It is also the first Noble Truth in Buddhism and the foundation of the Four Noble Truths, which are *duḥkha* (suffering), *duḥkha-samudaya* (the cause of suffering), *duḥkha-nirodha* (the end of suffering), and *duḥkha-nirodha-mārga* (the path to the end of suffering). To become awakened and free, it is necessary first to become aware of and understand this cycle of human existence. See also Ātman, Sukha.

गणेश
Gaṇeśa

Also Gaṇesha. From *gaṇa* ("multitude") and *īsha* ("lord"). Gaṇeśa is the son of Śiva and Pārvatī. According to legend, Pārvatī gave birth to her son Gaṇeśa while her husband Śiva was off hunting. Gaṇeśa was born fully mature, and immediately assumed the duty of protecting his mother. When Śiva returned to find Pārvatī naked, bathing, he also found this "stranger" in his home and promptly cut off Gaṇeśa's head. To his horror, he discovered that he had beheaded his own son, and promised Pārvatī that he would replace his son's head with the head of the first being he found. When he went outside, what he encountered first was an elephant, so he promptly took the head home and attached it to Gaṇeśa's body. He made Gaṇeśa, or Ganapati, the leader of his Army and decreed that everyone must pray to him before beginning any undertaking. Ganapati is beloved as the Lord of Categories: *gana* means "category," or "all that can be classified, comprehended, or quantified." Gaṇeśa embodies the relativity principle of the universe, through which the order of things and their relationships can be seen. He is also immensely popular as Vighneshvara (alternatively, Vighnaharta), Remover of Obstacles, the Deity of Beginnings, and the Deity of Wisdom. People pray to him for success when starting new ventures and business endeavors, hoping that he will bestow *siddhi* (powers of success) and *buddhi* (intelligence). His huge elephant head symbolizes wisdom, and his small, strong body suggests alacrity and might. From a philosophical point of view, his head is said to represent *brahman* (the Highest Reality), while his body represents *māyā* (illusion). His enormous ears are like "winnowing baskets" used to separate the real (*brahman*) from the unreal (*māyā*) with discrimination (*viveka*). Gaṇeśa has four hands: one carries a rope (to pull his devotees toward the truth), another wields an axe (to sever their attachments to material goods), and a third holds an Indian sweet called a *laddoo* (to reward them for their spiritual prowess); Gaṇeśa's fourth hand is always outstretched to offer his blessings. Gaṇeśa is also revered as the scribe who wrote down the beloved epic *Mahābhārata* (the story of the Bharat, or people of South Asia). See also MAHĀBHĀRATA, PĀRVATĪ, ŚIVA.

गुण
Guṇa

Three qualities, attributes, or characteristics of nature, or types of energy. These are:

Rajas रजस्

Vibrancy, activity, and passion; a state of motion and an overactive mind. From the verb root *raj* ("to glow"). *Rajas* also has pain in its nature, for pain arises from activity.

Tamas तमस्

Dormancy, dullness, inertia, and ignorance, a state in which the mind is underactive. From the verb root *tam* ("to perish").

Sattva सत्त्व

Luminosity, purity, harmony, and lightness, the balance of *rajas* and *tamas*, a balanced state wherein the mind can accurately discriminate. From the root *sat* ("being"), the present participle of *as* ("to be"). In contrast to *rajas, sattva* is a painless state, as it is a state where there is nothing to do, no desire, nowhere to go. All that remains is light and bliss.

The first of these motivates one to take action, to assert oneself, to be willful, to conquer, resist, and aspire. The second induces slothfulness, inertia, sleep, indifference, apathy, distintegration, and death. The third leads to harmonious living, well being, and equanimity. All of the *tri-guṇas*, or three *guṇas*, are believed to limit the soul, however, since they are driven by ego and motivated by desire, and also belong to the mental realm, which is by nature exclusive and divisive rather than inclusive and all-encompassing.

Guṇa also means "that which binds," since the three *gunas* also have the potential to stifle spiritual growth, binding one to the material world. *Rajas* binds man through ambition and drive, as does *tamas* through negligence and error, and *sattva* through virtue and knowledge for their own sake. The three *guṇas* are central to Ayurvedic science, as they provide a deeper understanding of our mental and spritiual nature than do the three biological humors (*vata*, *pitta*, and *kapha*) alone. In the *Bhaghavad Gītā*, Kṛiṣṇa teaches Arjuna to be a man of action, but reveals that in order to be spiritually liberated, one must move beyond the three *guṇas*, beyond human ego. Freedom over the power of the three *guṇas* is called *nistraiguna*, from *nir* ("without") plus *trai* ("three") and *guṇa* ("quality"). Only when one has gone beyond the three qualities of nature (*Trigunātitya*) can one surrender to the Divine and attain Oneness with God. See also Bhaghavad Gītā, Prakṛti.

गुरु
Guru

From the verb root *gri* ("to invoke," "to praise"), *guru* is also an adjective meaning "heavy," "weighty," "serious," or "venerable"—hence, "guru" literally means "heavy one." The word may also have a connection to the root *gur*, meaning "to raise," "lift up," or "make an effort." Its origins are in the *Guru Gītā*, the "song of the spiritual teacher" found in the *Mārkaṇḍeya Purāṇa*, a collection of mantras presented in the form of a dialog between Śiva and Pārvatī; in that context the root *gu* means "darkness" and *ru* means "removal." A guru is a spiritual guide and teacher who has attained enlightenment and who has the capacity to pass on his wisdom to others, illuminating the spiritual path, removing the darkness of ignorance, and shining the light of understanding.

Ideally, a guru also teaches his disciples, by example, how to live a good and ethical life; sadly, this is not in fact always the case.

In M. P. Pandit's translation of the *Kulārnava Tantra* (Chapter 13, Verse 104), an important Hindu Tantra text quoted in *The Yoga Tradition*, Śiva speaks to his wife Devī about the difficulty of finding a good guru: "There are many gurus, like lamps in house after house, but hard to find, O Devī, is the guru who lights up all like the sun." A classic example of the relationship between guru and *śisya* (pupil) is found in the *Bhagavad Gītā*, where Lord Kṛiṣṇa teaches the warrior Prince Arjuna to overcome his doubts and fears, ultimately attaining Godhood.

In addition to the outer guru (a separate person), there is also an inner guru—the higher self that can be known by developing our sense of inner listening, inner wisdom, and intuition. According to the *Vedas*, the inner guru is the most important source of knowledge. The practice of yoga ultimately connects one to this invaluable source of knowledge, peace, and strength. See also Bhagavad Gītā.

हंस

Haṃsa

The term *haṃsa* comes from the roots *ham*, meaning "expel," "abandon," or "release," and *sa,* meaning "to hold" or "to be." Considered an expression of the sound of the breath and of the rhythms of the universe, this word is closely related to the well-known mantra *Om.* This sound is the natural rhythm of the Self—the sound that occurs organically in the ebb and flow of the breath. Sanskrit tradition holds that we make this sound 21,600 times a day. In its complete form, *haṃsa* becomes *ahaṃsa,* meaning "I am He/She." This vibration can also be felt when inverting the syllables and repeating the phrase "*so' ham,*" which also means, "I am He/She": *so* is the inhalation, and *ham* the exhalation. When we breathe deeply and quiet the mind, we can hear these sounds deep within ourselves. According to the *Sahajiya,* or Doctrine of Nature, this sound embodies the meeting of the self with the higher self. Removing the consonants from *so' ham* leaves the primordial sound *Om.* See also Om.

हठयोग

Haṭha Yoga

Thought to derive from the verb root "*hath*" ("to force" or "stick fast," "hold firmly"), "Haṭha Yoga" combines the words *ha* ("sun") and *tha* ("moon") with the word *yoga* ("union"). Haṭha Yoga is the "yoga of force"; it is a practice of steadfastly balancing the opposing energies of the body—sun and moon, male and female, yin and yang, hot and cold, light and dark, right and left—which makes it possible to yoke and unify these energies through *āsana* (physical postures), *prāṇāyāma* (breath control), meditation, and *mudrās* ("energy seals"). Haṭha Yoga activates and purifies the energy centers of the body, stilling the wanderings of the mind and creating equanimity and balance, perhaps even leading to *samādhi,* or union with the Divine, and the creation of a divine, immortal comprehension of eternal existence (*divya-deha*). See also Āsana, Aṣṭāṅga Yoga (Prāṇayama), Mudrā, Samādhi.

हठयोगप्रदीपिका
Haṭha Yoga Pradīpikā

"Light on the Union of the Sun and Moon" or "Light on Haṭha Yoga." This is the title of the authoritative practical treatise on Haṭha Yoga authored by Yoga Swāmi Svātmarama in the mid-fourteenth century. In this work, Swāmi Svātmarama credits Matsyendra (Lord of the Fishes) and Gorakśa (an early preceptor of Haṭha Yoga) as being the teachers from whom he directly received the teachings of yoga. In his preface to the 1914 edition, yoga master Pancham Sinh states that there are two classes of yoga students: (1) those who study it theoretically; and (2) those who combine the theory with practice. He maintains that yoga is of very little use if studied theoretically, and that it was never meant for such a study. "In its practical form, however," he comments, "the path of the student is beset with difficulties." To offset these, modern students often turn to this ancient manual, which is as practical today as it was thousands of years ago. The *Haṭha Yoga Pradīpikā* offers 389 *floras* (verses) elucidating *haṭha vidya* (the science of Haṭha Yoga) and explaining the elements of Haṭha Yoga as a means of developing inner consciousness and moving toward bliss and union with the higher self. It is divided into four sections: (1) *āsana* (yoga postures) and *yamas* (restraints) as seen in the *Yoga Sūtras* of Patañjali; (2) *kriyā* (cleansing rituals) and *prāṇāyāma* (breath-control exercises); (3) *mudrās* (energy seals) and *bandhas* (energy locks); and (4) *samādhi* (union or liberation). See also HAṬHA YOGA, PĀRVATĪ.

होली
Holī

Often referred to as the "festival of colors," Holī falls on the day after the first full moon in March. This celebration of good harvest, fertility, and the spring season also commemorates the immortal love of Radha and Kṛiṣṇa, as well as the story in Hindu mythology of the demon Holikā, who is forgiven for her sins before her death. On the eve of Holī, huge bonfires are lit to ward off evil spirits. In the morning, neighborhood streets fill with people running, laughing, and splashing brightly colored powders, water, and paint onto each other's white clothes. An uninhibited atmosphere is created, where people celebrate together regardless of caste, sex, age, or past grudges. The bright colors symbolize joy, energy, forgiveness, love, unity, and life. Dances, folk songs, and the exchange of sweets are all part of this festive day.

ईश्वरप्राणिधान
Īshvara Praṇidhāna

Praṇidhāna means "devotion" or "surrender" and *Īshvara* means "God," "the Divine," "Great Ruler," or "Higher Power" and comes from the verb *is* ("to rule"). *Praṇidhāna* is a vow taken by a *bodhisattva* to commit one's life to helping others achieve enlightenment or liberation. *Īshvara praṇidhāna* is the state in which one surrenders to the Absolute, giving up the ego and sense of individual self, and surrendering to a higher power in service of others. *Īshvara* is one of the five *niyamas* (inner practices) of Aṣṭāṅga Yoga, believed to still the fluctuations of the mind and ultimately lead to *samādhi*. Practicing *īshvara praṇidhāna* helps still the mind insofar as when we recognize and embrace the realm of the Divine and connect with Source power, we automatically move away from the realm of the individual self, the ego, and all the afflictions, suffering, and separation that the ego-identity creates. When we do this, we realize we are not separate from the Divine or others, and begin to take our place in the great stream of life. See also Aṣṭāṅga Yoga, Kriya Yoga.

जैन

Jaina

Relating to the *jinas* ("victors," "conquerors"). The spiritual tradition of Jainism is, with Hinduism and Buddhism, one of the three major socioreligious movements in India. It was established in the sixth century B.C.E. by the charismatic ascetic Vardhamāna Mahāvīra (the "Great Hero"), who was a contemporary of Gautama Buddha. The twenty-four teachers of Jainism were called "conquerors," with Vardhamāna being the last in the line of a succession of teachers known as *tīrthankaras* ("ford-makers") that began with Riṣabha, who reportedly lived for 8.4 million years. Vardhamāna's work in shaping the philsophy of Jainism was undoubtedly influenced by the work of these "ford-makers." The Jainas believe that all beings may become liberated, blissful, and omniscient due to their own efforts, by following the teachings and actions of their spiritual teachers and through penance (*tapas*), renunciation, and adherence to a strict moral code. One of the main influences of this religion is the ethical precept of the practice of nonviolence (*ahimsā*). Another is the teaching of the laws of cause and effect (karma). The Jainist doctrine of *Syādvāda* posits that since every assessment of reality is subject to different conditions and limitations, it is possible that many different assessments of reality are simultaneously true. Thus, the Jainist view of reality is multifaceted and allows for many perspectives. This practical, down-to-earth religion holds that since all beings have souls, liberation is available to anyone. Thousands of years ago, Vardhamāna wandered India preaching his philosophy, naked but for a coat of ash. These days, *sādhu* can still be seen emulating this practice. See also Bhakti Yoga.

जीव
Jīva

From the root verb *jīv* ("to live" or "continue breathing"), this is the individual self, the embodied soul, the eternal, conscious omnipresent entity. In the yoga tradition, the soul is passive and unchanging. Tradition holds that enlightenment is attained when the *jīva* eradicates ignorance (*avidyā*) and stills the fluctuations of the mind (*vṛtti*). Another word for *jīva* is *puruṣa* ("what lies in the citadel of the body").

जीवनमुक्त
Jīvanmukta

Meaning "someone who is liberated in this lifetime," this word derives from the verb roots *much* and *mokś*—"to liberate," and *jīvan*—"living." Many spiritual traditions believe that it is possible to achieve enlightenment while still within the physical body. The body is not incompatible to enlightenment, according to Advaita Vedānta. Enlightenment occurs when ignorance (*avidyā*) has been eradicated. Fundamentally, the body, too, is seen as an illusion. Since the body is neither real nor unreal, it is not an obstacle to liberation. The *jīvanmukta* lives in his or her body, but is not of it. Also, the related word *jīvanmukti* means "a state of living liberation."

ज्ञान
Jñāna

Pronounced *gyāna*. From the root *jñā* ("to know"), this term means "knowledge," "wisdom," "understanding," "comprehension." In the Advaita Vedānta tradition, *jñāna* is the path to liberation or union with God. According to Jainism, it is the knowledge of worldly things.

SANSKRIT FACTS & LEGENDS

The sounds of the Sanskrit alphabet are considered the children of the primordial sound of the Absolute *Om*. All sounds derive from *Om*. In turn, they are called *matrikās* or "little mothers."

Sanskrit might have as many ways to say seer/sage/spiritual master as the Inuit language has for "snow." Among them are: *ṛiṣi, sādhu, guru, ṣrī, avatār, mahātman, ācārya, swāmi, sannyāsin, yogī,* and *yoginī.*

The potency of Sanskrit is so great that there is even a Tantric initiation ritual in which the teacher visualizes the letters of the Sanskrit alphabet in the adept's body and then makes them disintegrate until the student achieves union with God.

SANSKRIT FACTS & LEGENDS

A medieval scripture, the *Brihat-Samnyāsa Upaniṣad*, declares that if you chant *Om* 12,000 times, all your sins will disappear. If you chant *Om* 12,000 times a day for a year, you will enter the Godhead (*brahman*).

For a "dead language," Sanskrit is remarkably alive in the modern world. There is a village of 3,000 people in India who communicate only in the five-thousand-year-old language.

The *Mahābhārata* and the *Rāmāyana*, the two great Indian epics, were recited to a popular audience and passed down in the oral tradition by the Sūtas, who were not upper-class Brahmins. The two epics are thus composed in Classical Sanskrit mixed with local dialects, reflecting the men's natural speech rather than the more grammatically formal Sanskrit of Pāṇini.

ज्ञानयोग
Jñāna Yoga

Also Gyāna Yoga. The "yoga of wisdom." One of the Trimārga, or Threefold Path of Yoga, the triumvirate of classical yoga that also includes Bhakti Yoga and Karma Yoga. Often called the "Pathless Path," Jñāna Yoga is the "yoga of knowledge," based on the study of scripture, self-study, and direct inquiry, rather than following in the footsteps of a guru, performing a set system of beliefs or postures, or giving oneself over to the Divine through faith and devotion. In this, it is considered a yoga that develops the individual personality. In the Advaita Vedānta tradition, Jñāna Yoga is considered the path to the higher self (*ātman*) or liberation (*mokśa*). This freedom is gained through the individual's own efforts at study, questioning, and exploration. The *yogī* ultimately achieves the ability to distinguish the real from the unreal (*viveka*) and cultivates *vairagya* (nonattachment). When the soul has union with God based on wisdom, it can more easily overcome obstacles. When we see through the veil of illusion that surrounds us, we realize that the self is not distinct from the Divine. As we are already one with the Source, we need not look outside ourselves for the answers. See also Bhagavad Gītā, Bhakti Yoga, Karma Yoga.

कैवल्यपद
Kaivalyapad

Path of renunciation. "Aloneness," "isolation." This is a state of total detachment from matter and nature. It is a state of neither pain nor pleasure. In yoga, it is a state of liberation—a state of isolation that has been achieved through *viveka,* or discernment.

कालीदुर्गा
Kālī Durgā

From the root *kal*, "to incite" or "to impel," and *durgā,* which means "goddess" or "supreme female godhead." Kālī Durgā is "the black one," the malevolent form of the Goddess Devi/Pārvatī; Durgā is the fierce element of the cosmic duality. The name may be derived from the word *kālī*, which means "black," and *kāla*, which means "time." Kālī is "black" as she is enveloped in darkness, shrouded in shadow. This Goddess, who has a hundred different names, is considered the embodiment of past, present, and future time. She represents the destructive forces of nature—a necessary counterpoint to the creative elements of the universe. She is depicted as a fierce-looking, half-naked, wild-haired, wrathful warrior. A garland of skulls, one for each letter of the Sanskrit alphabet (the letters embody the sound of the Divine), adorns her chest like a macabre necklace. Her four arms wave in a powerful dance. One hand holds a severed head, another brandishes a machete-like weapon called a *kartri*, another dispels fear, and another gives ecstasy. She is sometimes depicted dancing atop the corpse of Lord Śiva, her consort, whose corpse represents the end of finite existence. Though feared by some, she is also worshipped and adored by *Bhairavas*, a Tantric sect called the "Fearless Ones," who understand that it is necessary to destroy that which is no longer productive, thus making room for creation. Without destruction, there can be no creation, and vice versa. See also DEVĪ, PĀRVATĪ, ŚIVA.

कलियुग
Kali Yuga

This phrase refers to an age of moral and spiritual decline, and derives from the roots *yuj* ("to unite," "union") and *kal* ("to incite," "to count or impel"). In this sense, *kali* does not refer to the Goddess Kālī but rather to "the losing throw of a die." There are said to be four *yuga*, or ages: *satya, treta, dvapara,* and the last and final age, *kali.* This is the age in which truth (the "cow of *dharma*"; the animal that represents the universe) has deteriorated to the point where it is standing on only one of its four legs. In the present day, we are believed to be in the dark age of *kali yuga.*

कर्म
Karma

From the root *kṛ* ("to act," "do," "make"), the term encompasses the meanings of "action," "deed," "rite," and "cause and effect." According to the laws of *karma*, our current situation in this life is the result of past actions in previous lifetimes. One's deeds in a past or current lifetime determine one's fate: in other words, "What goes around comes around." Repercussions will be carried over into the next lifetime until the cycle is complete—that is, when all karmic debts have been paid and one can reach nirvana. As Kṛiṣṇa says in the *Bhagavad Gītā*, "There are two paths on which the soul of both man (*manuṣya*) and God walk. The first path helps free it from the cycle of life and death. The second path is ascribed to cycles of rebirth and death according to deeds (karma)."

कर्मयोग

Karma Yoga

The "yoga of action"; "devotion to duty." Part of the Trimārga, or Threefold Path of Yoga—the triumvirate of classical yoga that also includes Bhakti Yoga and Jñāna Yoga—Karma Yoga is the yoga of awareness of our actions and their consequences. Also known as the "yoga of doing," it is fundamentally the yoga of service, and is based on the idea that our kinship with humanity is made concrete when we serve others selflessly, offering our skills, resources, time, energy, or entire lives to helping others without regard to recognition, outcome, or personal gain. Karma Yoga can take the form of charity work, volunteer service, selfless teaching, or other avenues of unconditional giving. Since the world is "the body of God," when we heal the world, we heal ourselves. This is one form of yoga that transcends schools and disciplines. *Yogīs* of all persuasions can follow this path. See also Bhagavad Gītā, Bhakti Yoga, Jñāna Yoga, Rāja Yoga.

क्लेश
Kleśa

From the root *klish, kleśa* means "to suffer" or "be in distress." This word means affliction, suffering, pain. There are five *kleśas,* or root causes, of human suffering. They are: *avidyā,* or ignorance; *asmitā,* or ego; *rāga,* or attachment; *dveṣa,* or aversion; and *abhiniveśa,* or the will to live.

कोश
Kośa

Also *kosha*. From the root *kuś*, "to unfold," the term also means "sheath," "layer," "subtle body," or "treasury." Three thousand years ago, the *kośas* were first written about in the *Upaniṣads* as a kind of roadmap of the inner landscape. There are five layers of subtle energy that envelop the individual from the periphery of the physical body to the center, or innermost core. Each sheath exists inside another, and as they are peeled away like the layers of an onion, energies become more and more subtle until the center sheath—the layer of bliss (*ānanda-maya kośa*)—is reached. The *anna-maya kośa* is often referred to as the *sthula-śarīra*, the "gross body" while the next three layers are considered the *suksma-śarīra* (the "subtle body"). In yoga practice, we seek to shift our awareness gradually from outer to inner. The sheaths of the body (from the outer layer inward) are:

Anna-maya kośa अन्नमयकोश
The physical body, or food sheath. This is the layer of skin, muscle, tissue, and bone. Expression is through

movement and the workings of the body (such as digestion and elimination).

Prāṇā-maya kośa प्राणामयकोश
The vital body, or breath sheath. This is the layer of the circulation of the breath and of life-force energy. Expression is through the breath and movement of energy.

Mano-maya kośa मनोमयकोश
The mental body, or sheath of the mind. This is the mental layer, encompassing the nervous system. Expression is through thought patterns.

Vijñāna-maya kośa विज्ञानमयकोश
Consciousness, or the sheath of intellect. This is the layer of higher states of awareness, or the "wisdom self." Expression is through observation or awareness. This is known as "witness consciousness," or the ability to stand outside the self and watch the fluctuations of mind, body, and breath objectively, observing them without judgment or attachment, as a witnessing awareness.

Ānanda-maya kośa आनन्दमयकोश
The sheath of bliss. This is the subtle core, the innermost layer where we exist purely in the moment, without thought, sensation, or judgment. Rather than

"feeling" such states as bliss, wholeness, integration, contentment, joy, and love, we embody them, and simply *are* them.

कृपालु
Kṛipālu

From *kṛpā*—"grace" or "favor. " The three types of grace are:

Sādhana-kṛpā साधनकृपा
Grace arising from individual effort.

Guru-kṛpā गुरुकृपा
Grace arising from the guidance of a teacher or master.

Divya-kṛpā दिव्यकृपा
Divine grace arising from union with God.

Kṛipālu is also the name of a style of yoga that focuses on body sensing and awareness, and of a famous yoga center in Massachusetts.

कृष्ण
Kṛiṣṇa

Also Krishṇa. From either *krṣ*, meaning "black," "dark," or *krṣ*, meaning "truth," and *na*, "bliss." Lord Kṛiṣṇa is also called "the Dark One," as dark blue and black were considered the colors of the infinite in ancient India. Kṛiṣṇa is the eighth incarnation of Viṣṇu and is considered an *avatār*, a Deity who has "crossed or passed over" to earth. (*Avatārs* are individual forms of the Supreme Being who descend from the spiritual realm to the material realm to delight, teach, and protect humankind in times of need. Though they have individual missions, their main purpose is to reveal the "Absolute Truth" and to remind humanity of its original state of bliss in the kingdom of God.)

Like Rāma, Kṛiṣṇa is revered for his bravery and ability to vanquish evil; it was Lord Kṛiṣṇa who delivered his sage battlefield advice to the warrior Arjuna in the *Bhaghavad Gītā*. Kṛiṣṇa is depicted playing a *muralī*, or Indian flute, symbolizing the "music of love" that is a source of joy for both humanity and the gods. He is also depicted with Rādha, his consort and devotee. Together, they represent the love shared between the human and the Divine. Kṛiṣṇa has 1,008 names, including Rādhā-Kṛiṣṇa. Another of his names is Govinda, from *go* ("cows") plus *inda* ("master") or, alternatively, from *go* ("speech") plus *vid* ("knower"). The literal meaning of this second possibility is "knower of the *Vedas*." This gentle cowherder was "learned in the *Vedas*, a master of speech, and a savior of the earth." Kṛiṣṇa is often depicted with his favorite cow. See also Rādhā, Viṣṇu.

क्रिया

Kriyā

"Action," "practice," "rite," "skill," "exercise," "movement," "function," "performance." *Kriyā* are traditional Haṭha Yoga purification rituals that awaken the *kuṇḍalinī* energy. These work on both gross and subtle levels to cleanse, replenish, and balance muscle tissue, bone matter, joints, blood, internal organs, the workings of the mind, and the subtle energies of the body. Though there are dozens of purification rituals, the six main ones are called *sat-kriyā.*

They are: *nauli* (abdominal churning to cleanse the intestines); *neti* (cleansing the nasal passages with water or string); *vasti* (cleansing the colon); *trātakam* (cleansing the eyes [the tear ducts] by gazing at an object without blinking); *kapālabhāti* ("skull-shining breath," or rapid diaphragmatic breath to cleanse the lungs); and *dhauti* (cleansing the stomach and rectum and teeth and throat). These ancient *kriyā* are still used by many *yogī* around the world to purify the body and mind and prepare them for higher consciousness.

क्रिया योग
Kriyā Yoga

The "active performance of yoga." This is the method of "yoga in action" outlined by Patañjali in the *Yoga Sūtras* more than two thousand years ago. It consists of three elements—"ascetic practice," "study and chanting of sacred hymns," and "dedication to the Lord of Yoga." These three pursuits are offered as a kind of performance guideline to the *yogī*, who will need diligence, guidance, and devotion on the arduous path to liberation. Chapter 11, Verse 1 of the *Yoga Sūtras* states: "Ascetic practice, study of sacred lore, and dedication to the Lord of Yoga is what constitutes the practice of Kriyā Yoga." Kriyā Yoga is considered an adjunct to the Eight Limbs of Yoga, or Aṣṭāṅga Yoga, which outlines the path to liberation through eight stages of yoga practice. See also AṢṬĀṄGA YOGA.

कुल
Kula

From the root *kul*—"grouping together." *Kula* means "group," "school," "clan," "cluster," or anything that is bound or contracted together by the forces of energy. It also denotes the human body, home, community, family, lineage, the world, the universe, the cosmos, and divine creative energy.

कुण्डलिनी शक्ति

Kuṇḍalinī Śakti

From the verb *kuṇḍ* ("to burn"), *kuṇḍalinī* means "serpent" or "life-force." It also means "coiled, winding, spiraled one," as this powerful life-force is considered a coiled goddess slumbering at the base of the spine. This primal cosmic energy, or *śakti*, sleeps in the *mūlādhāra* (root) chakra until the practice of yoga, including *prāṇāyāma*, meditation, mantra, or other spiritual pursuits awakens it. In other words, the *kuṇḍalinī* energy is a physical manifestation of the primordial creative cosmic energy, or *śakti*, coiled in the base of the spine of the human body. Once unbound, it then begins to travel up the *suṣumṇa nāḍi*, the central channel of energy in the body, and the *iḍā nāḍi* and *piṅgalā nāḍi*, activating the chakras. When it reaches the *sahasrāra* (crown) chakra at the top of the head—the highest point in the body—union with the Divine is attained. *Kuṇḍalinī śakti* is the mother of the primordial, pulsing sound of the universe within us, the original intelligent life-force that embodies creation, existence, and dissolution. It is the active power that gives birth to the universe and the universe within. The *Haṭha Yoga Pradīpikā* states, "You should awaken the sleeping serpent by grasping its tail."

Kuṇḍalinī śakti represents a very ancient teaching also found in Native American shamanic traditions. For example, Mayan elders refer to "kuthalini" as the coiled life-force that rises through the spine when a person is enlightened. Quetzalcoatl, the great spirit messenger of ancient Central America, is the name for the sleeping serpent residing at the base of the spine (coccyx) until awakened. Various shamanic traditions also use sweatlodges, trance dance, fasting, silence, prayer, and plant medicines to facilitate the awakening of *kuṇḍalinī*. See also CHAKRA, KUṆḌALINĪ YOGA, NĀḌI, ŚAKTI, ŚIVA.

कुण्डलिनीयोग
Kuṇḍalinī Yoga

A form of yoga that seeks to awaken the *kuṇḍalinī śakti* through set sequences of yoga *āsanas* (postures) and *prāṇāyāma* (breath control exercises). Typically, the breath-control exercises involve *anuloma-viloma* (alternate nostril breathing) to balance the *iḍā nāḍi* (left energy channel) and the *piṅgalā nāḍi* (right energy channel) and *kapalabhāti* ("breath of fire"), a rapid diaphragmatic breathing that helps to move energy up the *suṣumṇa nāḍi* (central energy channel). As the *kuṇḍalinī śakti* rises, it strikes each chakra and activates the energy there to bring about awakening, balance, and vibrancy. Ultimately, the *kuṇḍalinī* rises through all six chakras and enters the seventh, the *sahasrāra* (crown) chakra, the highest spiritual center of the body. Here the individual self merges with the universal self, and higher consciousness is attained. Kuṇḍalinī Yoga remained a secret discipline until 1969, when Yogī Bhajan, Ph.D., a master of White Tantric Kuṇḍalinī Yoga, taught the tradition to his disciples. See also CHAKRA, KUṆḌALINĪ ŚAKTI, NĀḌI, ŚAKTI, ŚIVA.

लययोग

Laya Yoga

The "yoga of dissolution." This is a form of Tantra Yoga in which the energies of the individual chakras are dissolved through the awakening and ascent of the *kuṇḍalinī śakti.* The passage of this once-dormant energy leads to dissolution (*laya*) of the ego. Lallā, the fourteenth-century Kashmiri mystic poet, holy woman, Sufi, *yogī*, and Śiva devotee who was popularly known as Lal Ded (b. 1326), wrote of her ecstatic union with Śiva through the practice of Laya Yoga: "I, Lallā, became enraptured in the bliss of ecstasy, through concentration and rhythmic recitation of Om. I worked hard to give the letter proper pitch and volume, and the effect was that I was set free, attaining enlightenment. That is; from ashes have I transformed into pure gold" (Vākya 1).

लीला
Līlā

"Divine play" or "sport." *Līlā* is a worldview in which creation is considered a drama conceived and realized by God for the sheer joy of it. The idea of a cosmic play is similar to Shakespeare's "All the world's a stage, and all the men and women merely players," with the added notion that Divine Sport is God's motivation for creating this world. As a child Kṛiṣṇa engaged in *līlā*. Kṛiṣṇa Līlā is celebrated every August on Kṛiṣṇa's birthday with greatly festive, creative, and colorful dance, song, and drama.

लिङ्ग

Liṅga

Also *liṅgam, lingam*. From "mark" or "sign," and meaning "phallus." In ancient India, the Aryan people worshipped sacred phalli as symbols of creation and the embodiment of the productive and regenerative power of the cosmos, which is manifest in all things great and small. The *liṅga* (phallus) is also a symbol of Lord Śiva and is thus often called "Śiva Liṅga," which rises from a *yoni* (vulva) base. This union of Śiva (male) and Śakti (nature/female) represents the meeting of the universal creative principle with the universal productive principle, symbolizing intercourse as cosmic union. See also Śakti, Śiva, Yoni.

लोक
Loka

"World," "universe," "plane," "realm." *Loka* can also mean "a state of light," "heaven," or "the ascension of the soul." Indian culture traditionally holds that there are seven planes or plateaus of the universe, built by the Supreme Being to represent the heavens, light, and becoming. They are *bhūrloka*, the material world (from *bhū*—earth); *bhūvarloka*, the world of becoming (from *bhū*—to become); *svarloka*, the world of light (from *svar*—heaven); *maharloka*, the infinite world (from *mahas*—vastness); *janaloka*, the world of joy of spiritual living (from *jan*—to be born); *taparloka*, the world of Will or Conscious Force (from *tapas*—spiritual force/fire); and *satyaloka*, the world of the highest truth of being (from *satya*—truth). In the human body, these *loka* are said to exist in the feet, genitals, navel, heart, throat, third eye, and crown of the head.

महाभारत
Mahābhārata

This beloved Indian tale, meaning "The Great Bhārata," describes a war between two rival families, the Pāṇḍavas and the Kauravas, and imparts many ethical, philosophical, and moral lessons about virtue and selflessness, karma and liberation. The *Mahābhārata* is based on popular stories of kings, gods, seers, and sages. It was created in India's preclassical, or epic, age, from about 1000 to 100 B.C.E., and was passed down orally by priests, wandering mendicants, ascetics, actors, and minstrels who recited, danced, sang, and performed the tale. These various stories were unified in 350 C.E. into a 100,000-verse sacred text, written in Sanskrit and disseminated throughout India by royalty and wealthy patrons of the arts. It is still extremely popular today, and is performed all over the world.

In this ancient epic, a king has two sons. The elder, Dhritarashitra, is blind, so the younger, Pāṇḍu, succeeds to the throne after the king's death. King Pāṇḍu has five sons, while his blind brother Dhritarashitra has one hundred sons, the Kauravas. Pāṇḍu's eldest son Duryodhana begins to resent his father's love of the Pāṇḍavas, and tricks the Pāṇḍavan Prince Yudhishthira into gambling away his kingdom and wife in a game of dice. The five Pāṇḍava brothers are then banished. After a thirteen-year exile, the virtuous brothers return and demand the restoration of their kingdom. The hundred Kaurava brothers choose to fight instead. As the kin battle it out, Lord Kṛiṣṇa must descend to earth to try to restore law and order. After eighteen days of battle, the Kauravas are defeated.

The *Mahābhārata* contains the earliest complete work on yoga, the *Bhagavad-Gītā*, in which Kṛiṣṇa lectures the reluctant warrior Arjuna on the nature of ethical action, just prior to a battle in which he must take up arms against his own kin. This beloved epic, together with the *Rāmāyaṇa*, deeply informs the Hindu culture of India. See also Bhagavad Gītā.

महत्
Mahat

From the root *mahā*, meaning "great," "supreme,"

"mighty," "powerful," "noble." *Mahat* is the great principle of nature; cosmic intelligence.

महात्मन
Mahātman

Also Mahātma महात्म. This word also derives from *mahā* ("great"), plus *ātman* ("self"). The meaning is essentially "supreme soul" or "great self." It is used as an honorific for outstanding individuals, such as Mohandas K. Gandhi, often called Mahātma Gandhi.

महायान
Mahāyāna

From *mahā* ("great") and *yāna* ("vehicle"). Literally, the "Greater Ox-Cart," meaning "Higher Vehicle," or "vehicle to a higher state." Before Mahāyāna Buddhism arrived in India in the first century C.E., the most popular form of Buddhism was Theravada, which centered on the Eightfold Noble Path and required its disciples to follow this path through the rigors of meditation. Since the majority of people could not follow the strict practices of Theravada, a more populist form of Buddhism was created, descending from the same stream of thought as the first Buddha (Gautama, or Siddhārtha). They called their new religion the "Greater Ox-Cart," since it had the potential to carry people from all stations and classes to enlightenment. *Mahāyāna* offered enlightenment for the many, rather than for the few, and presented the idea of levels of Buddhahood attained in various lifecycles or incarnations. The concept of the *bodhisattva*, or "Buddha-in-waiting," was central to this doctrine. A *bodhisattva* gave up his worldly life to be of service to the Buddha, teaching others the tenets of Buddhism and acting with great compassion, selflessness, and virtue to all he encountered. Mahāyāna Buddhism held that one of these *bodhisattvas* could be the "Second Coming of Buddha," the Maitreya who would heal the world. See also BODHISATTVA, BUDDHA, DUḤKHA, MAITREYA.

मैत्रेय

Maitreya

"Friendly," "benevolent," "loving"; also refers to the Mahāyāna Buddhist belief in the "Future Buddha," the "Second Coming" of Buddha, who would arrive on earth and enlighten the world. As the coming of this *maitreya* was prophesized by the First Buddha (Guatama Buddha), Mahāyāna philosophy holds that the "Future Buddha" must already be among us, going through the cycle of karma and assuming various incarnations. According to this thought, anyone could be the Maitreya—the beggar, the saint, the child—we all contain the potential to be holy. In Buddhism, the qualities of *maitreya* are represented by the "Laughing Buddha," a fat, jolly, smiling Buddha found throughout Asia, often gracing shop entrances. His protruding belly is a symbol of happiness, luck, and generosity. In Japan, the Laughing Buddha is called Hotei; he is one of the "seven lucky gods" and carries a sack full of candy and other goodies on his back, and shares his benevolence and wealth with all he meets on the path of life. See also BUDDHA, MAHĀYĀNA.

मैत्री
Maitrī

Friendliness, love. One of the highest virtues in yoga, a quality inherent in all enlightened beings and *bodhisattvas*. In Miller's translation of the *Samādhi Pada*, Patañjali states: "Through cultivation of friendliness (*maitrī*), compassion (*karunā*), joy (*muditā*), and indifference (*upekṣā*) to pleasure and pain, virtue and vice respectively, consciousnesss becomes favorably disposed, serene and benevolent." In the *Vibhūti Pada*, Patañjali writes: "He gains moral and emotional strength by perfecting friendliness (*maitrī*) and other virtues towards one and all."

माला
Mālā

A garland or string of beads used for prayer when reciting mantras, like a rosary. It has 108 beads, one for each of the earthly desires to be transcended.

मंडल
Mandala

From the Sanskrit word for "circle," "connection," "community." It also means "entire world," "center of the Universe," "magic circle," or "healing circle." A mandala is a sacred symbol used for meditation, particularly in the Tibetan Buddhist tradition. Though there are many kinds of mandalas, they are typically vibrant, colorful representations of the whole world, with an enlightened being residing in the center. As one meditates on a mandala, one's consciousness passes through outer protective circles (symbolizing grasping at the surface or exterior of things), then enters square structures and inner gates that enclose the center point or *bindu* (which symbolizes the essence of life), considered the palace of Buddha. These sacred symbols have individual characteristics representing the distinct qualities of the particular deities they house. Though mandalas can be made of many materials, and can even refer to a geographic location or a space visualized in the mind, some of the most intricate are sand mandalas painted by Tibetan Buddhist monks, wherein the process of creation itself is no less important than the actual mandala. Monks train in their art for years, undergoing a series of rituals, purifications, and rites to consecrate body and mind, only to have these beautiful works blown away instantaneously in a gust of wind. Such is the impermanent nature of existence, and the sand is believed to carry its illuminated essence back to nature. Many traditions in Western culture have their own sacred circles, like the medicine wheels used in Native American healing ceremonies and the talismans of blessing and protection found in many other religions and traditions. Mandalas differ from *yantras* in that these separate entitites representing holy abodes tend to be far more complex in design and liturgical representation than *yantras*, which are physical expressions of divine sound vibration, or mantras. See also MANTRA, YANTRA.

मन्त्र

Mantra

From the verb *man* ("to think") and *tra*, meaning "instrumental," the *mantra* is a word, phrase, or hymn with sacred or spiritual resonance, significance, or value, or "that which brings thoughts together." The literal meaning is "instrument of thought"; this suggests that a mantra is a vehicle by which higher consciousness is manifest—a means by which we become harmonious with the world. Mantras raise consciousness, quieting and elevating one's state of mind. Sanskrit words form the basis for sacred mantras, and each one of the letters of the Sanskrit alphabet (called *matrikās*, or "little mothers") is believed to constitute the Divine in the form of sound (*śabda brahman*, or Supreme Sound). This "soundless sound" is believed to exist in all things in the universe and can be activated with the deeply resonant vibration of mantra that connects us to all living things. The belief that these sacred Sanskrit sounds can activate divine energy within the human (*jīvan*) is reflected in the fact that the letters of the Sanskrit alphabet are depicted in ancient *yantras*, mandalas, and diagrams as embedded in the petals of the chakras, the energy centers in the human body.

There are a myriad of different mantras, reportedly as many as 70,000. They can be male (solar), or gender-neutral. Female, or lunar, mantras are also known as *vidyas*. One-syllable mantras are called *bija mantras*; the word *bīja* means "seed," and these sounds contain the essence or seed of the Divine. The best known *bīja mantra* is *Om.* There are also string or garland mantras, like those in the Chants section at the back of this book, and unspoken mantras (*ajapa,* the sound of the in-and-out breath, or *hang-sah*). There are also mantras that are written down (*likhita*) as a spiritual practice, in much the same way that *sūtras* are copied mindfully as a form of meditation.

Though mantras are evoked for their deep vibratory and healing effect on consciousness and energy, in ancient times, they often served more practical purposes, such as warding off evil or disease. Later, mantra recitation, called *japa* (literally, "whispering") developed as a ritual wherein a disciple is given a secret mantra by his guru (a *ṛiṣi* who had received the mantra directly from Source during meditation). This mantra may or may not have a literal meaning, but it contains the pure vibration of divine power, which is also passed down to the student through the sound. Mantra Yoga, the "science of sound," uses the repetition or recitation of a mantra as the path to liberation (*mokśa*). In Mantra Yoga, the inner sound (*nāda)* is awakened through the outer sound (*mantra*). Nowadays many *yogī* continue this ancient ritual by beginning and/or ending their yoga practice with a mantra to evoke the Divine, to offer themselves and their practice to a higher power, and to express gratitude to a teacher and acknowledge his or her lineage. These mantras can be ancient quotations from the *Vedas* or other scriptures; prayers to the Gods; prayers for peace and happiness of all beings; or personal prayers offered in sound and tone. See also the Chants section and entries CHAKRA, NĀDA YOGA, OM.

माया
Māyā

From the verb root *mā* ("to measure," "limit," "give form to"). *Māyā* is the veil of illusion that prevents human beings from perceiving the Divine. It is also sometimes defined as "that which measures." In Advaita Vedānta, it is considered "that which causes the illusory nature of the universe." There are two aspects of this veil: *avidyā māyā*—the ignorance that separates man from God; and *vidyā māyā*, the wisdom that eventually allows man to become liberated, thus joining with God in Divine union.

मोक्ष
Mokśa

From the verb *mokś* ("to liberate"), this term means "spiritual freedom" or "release" and is considered human beings' ultimate goal—to be released from the bonds of ignorance and suffering. In yoga, *mokśa* is the culmination of Aṣṭāṅga, the Eight-limbed Path to Enlightenment, the aim of which is the achievement of *samādhi*. See also Aṣṭāṅga Yoga, Samādhi.

मुद्रा
Mudrā

From *mud* ("joy") and *rā* ("to give"). "Hand pose," "seal," "stamp." *Mudrās* are called "energy seals" because they seal (*mudrānāt*) the energy of the universe in the body, leading to a higher state of consciousness. In the yoga tradition, *mudrās* are a way of holding the *prāṇa* within the body in a beneficial way, and of healing, cleansing, and activating physical and spiritual release. They are used as rituals, offerings, salutations, means of meditation, and means of encouraging specific energetic effects on the different *kośas* (layers) of the body. They are also used to channel the breath and energy in meditation. There are dozens of *mudrās,* and while we often think of *mudrās* as hand gestures, there are also whole-body *mudrās*, like the *yoga mudrā* (gesture of understanding of nonduality) in which the benefits of the yoga practice are "sealed in" the body before completing the yoga practice.

Deities, saints, gods, and goddesses are often pictured with their hands in *mudrās*, making gestures of devotion or offering, and in classical Indian dance—which often recounts ancient myths and legends—the hands play an important part of the storytelling process, through their graceful and expressive movements. *Mudrās* also express feelings and convey meanings such as charity, knowledge, and courage, and one can offer a *mudrā* to a god, goddess, nature god, guru, teacher, friend, or even a complete stranger. Some powerful *hasta* (hand) *mudrās* are:

Añjali mudrā अञ्जलिमुद्रा

Añjali means "offering." This gesture of putting the fingertips together and joining the hands at the heart is often called "prayer pose." By joining the right and left hands together, we join the right and left sides of the brain and body, yoking them gently at the heart in a symbolic "shrine" or "steeple." When we make this gesture, we are "offering" ourselves from our deepest core—the heart chakra, whose "voice" speaks louder than the mind. In yoga, this *mudrā* is often accompanied by the Sanskrit greeting *namaste*—"the light/Divine within me greets the light/Divine within you"—which is uttered to give over one's practice as a devotional offering to a higher power. This gesture and greeting together underscore the yogic philosophy of seeing the Divine in everyone, of "hearts touching hearts" and meeting in a state of grace. *Añjali mudrā* is commonly used in India as a daily greeting or salutation, as we might say "hello" in the West.

Dhyāna mudrā ध्यानमुद्रा

"Gesture of meditation." *Dhyāna* means "meditation" and is one of the eight stages of yoga practice in Aṣṭāṅga Yoga, or the "Eight-limbed Path." This is a gesture used to deepen meditation, enhance awareness, and send the breath and *prāṇa* throughout the entire body. In this *mudrā*, which is done while sitting in a comfortable meditation pose with the spine straight and the chest wide and heart open, the right hand rests in the palm of the left hand at the lap, with the tips of the thumbs gently touching. In the yoga tradition, the right hand represents the sun, and the left hand, the moon. This symbolic hand gesture creates a circle of energy, balancing the body and the mind and awakening a deep unity within.

Jñāna mudrā ज्ञानमुद्रा

"Gesture of knowledge/wisdom." *Jñāna* means "knowledge" or "wisdom." Sitting in a comfortable meditation pose with the spine straight and the chest wide and heart open, here the arms rest on the thighs and the hands rest on the thighs or knees, palms facing up. The elbows are drawn in toward the torso. The tips of the index fingers touch the tips of the thumbs, while the little, ring, and middle fingers are extended. This is a gesture that slows the breath, increases blood flow to the brain, and connects us to higher knowledge and inner wisdom as we symbolically allow the individual self (represented by the index finger) to bow to and enter the realm of the universal self (represented by the thumb).

मुक्ति
Mukti

Liberation, release, spiritual freedom. From the verb root *much* and *mokś* ("to liberate"). *Mukti* refers to being liberated from bondage and/or the fetters of karma or material existence and attaining freedom and bliss. According to the great poet Rabindranath Tagore, *mukti* is "the one abiding ideal in the religious life of India," which he defines as "the deliverance of man's soul from the grip of self, its communion wih the Infinite Soul through its union in *ānanda* with the universe." Not merely a theological doctrine or something to be studied in a classroom, *mukti* is, according to Tagore, a larger "spiritual truth and beauty of our attitude toward our surroundings, our conscious relationship with the Infinite, and the lasting power of the Eternal in the passing moments of our life." For Tagore, who advocated an "open" school in nature, this ideal is made possible by living intimately with nature and by "growing in an atmosphere of service offered to all creatures, tending trees, feeding birds and animals, learning to feel the immense mystery of the soil and water and air." See also Jīvanmukta.

नादयोग
Nāda Yoga

The yoga, or union, of sound. *Nāda* means "sound" or "tone" and "universal pulse of life" or "flowing stream of consciousness." In yoga, *nāda* refers to the nasal sound often found in mystical words. *Yoga* means "union" or "path toward union." Nāda Yoga is an ancient, scientific practice that originated in India around 200 B.C.E., sprung from the Vedic tradition of Śabda Yoga (sound mysticism, the "yoga of sound"). It explores the relationship of sound to consciousness, using sound and rhythm as a path to healing, awareness, and spiritual understanding. Nāda Yoga stems from the belief that the primordial sound (*śabda)* is a root vibrational energy or force from which the ultimate reality springs. Everything in this world vibrates with this "sound within sound," including human beings, who embody this sound in the heartbeat. There are two types of nada—*āhata nāda*, or "struck sound" created by friction, and *anāhata nāda*, unstruck sound, which is the naturally occurring and eternal song of the earth and all beings. The heart chakra is called *anāhata chakra,* as it is the part of the body most connected to this sound. In Nāda Yoga, chanting sacred mantras attunes our inner rhythm to this ancient, primal pulse and connects us to this primordial singing beneath the surface of the world. Through chanting and drumming, we also harmonize the different frequencies in our bodies, tuning the chakras and balancing the right and left hemispheres of the brain. This synchronizes the body/mind, leading to relaxation, heightened creativity, and higher states of consciousness. See also CHAKRA, MANTRA, YANTRA.

नाडि

Nāḍi

Conduit; one of the approximately seventy-two thousand subtle channels of energy in the body through which *prāṇa* (life-force energy) circulates. *Nāḍi* are "cables" composed of three layers: the innermost (*sirā*), middle (*damanī*), and outer (*nāḍi*). The entire channel itself is also called a *nāḍi.* There are three main *nāḍi* in the body that connect the chakras, or energy centers. They are:

Suṣumṇa nāḍi सुषुम्णा नाडि
"Very gracious channel." This is the central channel of energy in the body, running alongside or parallel to the spine, where the *kuṇḍalinī śakti* (serpent energy) moves, activating the chakras as it threads its way up to the top of the head. *Mokśa* (liberation) is attained when the *kuṇḍalinī* reaches the crown chakra, joining the individual self with the Higher Power in bliss.

Iḍā nāḍi इडा नाडि
"Pale channel." This is the conduit for *prāṇa* on the left side of the central channel. It affects the parasympathetic nervous system (regulating "rest and digest") and is calming and cooling when activated. It is the carrier of female, lunar energy throughout the body.

Piṅgalā nāḍi पिंगला नाडि
"Red-colored channel." This is the conduit for *prāṇa* on the right side of the central channel. It affects the sympathetic nervous system (regulating the "fight or flight" response) and is warming, energizing, and invigorating when activated. It transports the masculine, solar energy throughout the body.

नमस्ते
Namaste

From *na* ("not"), *ma* ("mine"), and *te* ("to you"). The literal meaning is "honor/obeisance" (*namas*) to you (*te*). Also translated as literally meaning "Not mine, but Thine—Yours, the Divine." This phrase is variously translated as "The light in me greets the light in you" or "The Divine in me recognizes the Divine in you." This is the traditional, everyday greeting in India—with fingertips touching and hands held at the heart in *añjali mudrā*. This expression is often used in yoga classes to begin or complete the practice, offering one's soul to the Divine. It is also often used in the context of worship. See also MUDRĀ.

नेतिनेति
Neti-neti

From the word *na* ("not") and *iti* ("thus"). "Not thus, not thus" or "not such, not such" or "not this, not this." In the *Upaniṣads*, Yajñavalkya said, "The Ātman is not thus, not thus," expressing the belief that the *ātman*, or higher reality, is beyond definition. It is neither this nor that, and cannot be put into words. In Vedantic philosophy, the entire material plane is considered an illusion, and all the veils of illusion must be stripped away to reveal the essential self. In other words, true reality is "not this, not this"—we are not our roles in society or family, our jobs, our accomplishments, our bodies, our egos, our minds. We are our essential, highest selves, that which defies definition, that which exists beyond material, individual reality.

निरोध
Nirodha

"Control," "restraint," "restriction," "cessation." *Nirodha* forms the basis of the last three of the Eight Limbs of Yoga: *dhāraṇa* (concentration), *dhyāna* (meditation), and *samādhi* (pure contentment, enlightenment, bliss). One of the most famous aphorisms of the *Yoga Sūtras* is "*Citta vritti nirodha,*" which is translated as "restricting the fluctuations of the mind" or "controlling the fluctuations of thought"—this is the key to reaching nirvana. *Vritti* comes from the verb root *vṛt*—"to turn, revolve, move." Stilling the mind, however, is by no means an easy thing to do. As the warrior Arjuna says to Kṛiṣṇa in the *Bhagavad Gītā*, "The mind is very restless, forceful, and strong. It is more difficult to control the mind than to control the wind." See also Aṣṭāṅga Yoga, Yoga Sūtra.

निर्वाण

Nirvāṇa

From the roots *vā* ("to blow") and *nir* ("out"), *nirvāṇa* literally means "to blow out (from lack of fuel)." It is extinction, perfection, the Great Peace, absolute freedom, and unconditional *tathatā,* or "suchness." Nirvana is considered a state of enlightenment because, when it is reached, all the impressions or imprints of karma have been extinguished and one is free from the wheel of karma. This state of bliss is believed, in the yoga tradition, to be achieved when the mind has been controlled to the point of utter stillness. The

Mokśa-Dharma, the twelfth book of the *Mahābhārata*, states, "Yoked by that joy, he delights in the practice of meditation. Thus do the *yogins* go to nirvana, free from ill." See also SAṂSĀRA.

निवृत्तिमार्ग
Nivritti-mārga

From the roots *vri* ("to turn") and *ni* ("back"). This is the path of renunciation, or turning one's back on the world of material things, turning away from the world. In the *Bhagavad Gītā*, *dharma*, or duty, is composed of two parts: taking an active stand in the world (*pravritti*) and backing away from activity (*nivritti*). Thus, the fallow periods and the periods of cultivation and harvest are equally important aspects of liberation.

ओजस्
Ojas

From the verb root *jas* ("strength"), *ojas* means "vitality," "spiritual energy," "radiance," "magnificence." It is used to refer to the seminal fluids that are converted into subtle energy through yoga when stored in the body through the practice of *brahmacharya* (chastity).

The term *ojas* is used in Āyurveda for a highly refined substance that is converted into a subtle energy. This energy specifically prevents the decay and fragmentation of the mind and body and provides strength against all disease. The Bengali commentator and medicinal writer Cakrapanidatta (eleventh century C.E.) describes two types of *ojas*: *para* and *apara*. *Para ojas* is located in *hridaya* (the heart) and occurs in the quantity of *ashta bindu* (eight drops); *apara ojas* is located in the *dasa dhamanīs* (ten vessels) originating from the heart. According to Suśruta, the father of Ayurvedic surgery, *ojas* is viscous, slightly yellow, slimy, cold, and sweet in taste. *Ojas* circulates throughout the entire human being and is responsible for natural immunity against physical and mental disease; its loss from the body leads to decay and disease.

ॐ

Om

The *prāṇava*, the Eternal. This is the primordial Sanskrit sound (*prāṇava*), the One sacred sound from which all word variations originate. Considered the "sound of all sounds" because it originates from the sounds of nature and embodies them in its vibration, this mystical single-syllable word and its Sanskrit symbol represent the Divine Presence and Power that is the Universe. Two thousand years after the sound of *Om* was discovered by *ṛiṣis* in ancient India, an anonymous sage explained the three parts of the mantra in the *Māṇḍūkya Upaniṣad*. He wrote, "'Aum' consists of four, not three elements . . . the fourth is soundless: unutterable, a quieting down of all the differentiated manifestations, blissful, peaceful, nondual. . . . " In the metaphysical terms of Advaita Vedānta, the three sounds of the mantra A-U-M reflect the three divinities—inner, outer and superconscient.

When making the sound, there are the sounds of ah, oh, mmm, and silence. In the yoga treatise *Gorakśa-Paddhati* ("Tracks of Gorakśa"), which may have been written in the twelfth or thirteenth centuries, *Om* does symbolize the Absolute, but its parts (A-U-M) represent the earth (*bhūh*), middle region (*bhūvah*), and heaven (*svah*).

As Patañjali states in the *Yoga Sūtras*, "When Aum reveals itself, introspection is attained and obstacles fall away." *Om*, also called *Omkāra*, is usually chanted at the beginning of ceremonies, as a prelude to mantras, and before and after yoga practice as an offering to the Divine. Chanting *Om* can create a shift in consciousness, as it represents the passage of birth, life, death, and rebirth, and the resonance is said to activate the seven chakras. It has been noted that the word "Aum" bears a resemblance to the Hebrew word "amen" often used at the end of Jewish blessings and prayers to acknowledge the Divine. One beautiful definition of *Om* is "summoning God." See also HAṂSA, MANTRA.

ॐ तत् सत्
Om Tat Sat

This is a sacred expression meaning "Thou Art That." It denotes that we are the Divine, and that we should look within ourselves to find the holy. It embodies the meaning and power of *Om* (the vibration of creation), *tat* (the radiance or light perceived in deep meditation); and *sat* (higher consciousness). See also OM, SAT, TAT.

पद्म
Padma

Lotus, the Goddess. In Buddhist iconography, the Buddha is always depicted sitting on a lotus leaf. The lotus is said to represent the power of transformation, as its roots take hold in a muddy swamp and yet the flower blossoms into a thing of great beauty and luminescence. So, too, can the self transcend its humble origins and rise above them to achieve a state of radiant bliss and enlightenment. In meditation and in yoga, the Lotus posture or *Padmāsana*, is one of the most widely practiced of all the *āsanas*, embodying the nobility and grace of this ethereal flower. For that reason, this representative posture is called the "Royal posture" or "Throne of the Lotus flower." The subtle energy centers of the body, the chakras, are also called lotuses (*padma*), due to their swirling, circular form and the way that the life-force energy (*prāṇa*) flows to and from them. Finally, the lotus is also a symbol of the feminine principle or *yoni*, or vulva/womb. See also BUDDHA, CHAKRA, PRĀṆA, YONI.

परमात्मन्
Paramātman

From *parama* ("highest") and *ātman* ("self"). This is the supreme self, the Absolute. It refers to the singular transcendental self *(paramātman).* The self that exists in myriad forms and beings is called *jīvātman* ("liberated higher self").

पार्वती
Pārvatī

Literally, "daughter of the mountain." Pārvatī is Lord Śiva's consort. It was Pārvatī who is credited with helping spread knowledge of yoga in the world. Once, when Śiva and Pārvatī were on a deserted island together, Śiva explained to his consort the mysteries of yoga. A fish overheard their conversation, and when Śiva discovered him eavesdropping, he sprinkled water on him and gave him divine form. The Lord of The Fishes (*Matsyendra*) then disseminated yoga throughout the land and became the teacher to Gorakśa, who was an early teacher of Haṭha Yoga in the tenth to eleventh centuries. While Pārvatī is generally thought of as Śiva's consort, some schools of thought hold that these deities are in fact neither male nor female, but instead represent particular aspects of an individual God. In this viewpoint, Pārvatī represents the "mother" aspect of Lord Śiva, as she is considered the "Divine Mother" or the "Mother Goddess." This beautiful Goddess embodies the wife and mother archetype, symbolizing blissful matrimony (to Śiva) and contented motherhood (of

Gaṇeśa). Alone, she is depicted riding on a lion, the Queen of the Jungle. She is also often portrayed with Śiva and Gaṇeśa as part of the Divine Family, which makes its home on Mount Kailasa in the Himalayas. Pārvatī's "natural" family tree consists of some of the great wonders of the Indian landscape: she is beloved as a daughter of the magnificent Himalayan mountains and sister to the sacred Ganges River. She also assumes several other divine forms, among them the fierce warrior goddesses Durga ("Goddess Beyond Reach") and Kālī ("Goddess of Destruction"). She is also called Uma. See also DEVĪ, GAṆEŚA, KĀLĪ DURGĀ, ŚIVA.

पतञ्जलि
Patañjali

The author, about two thousand years ago, of the *Yoga Sūtras*. Details about Patañjali's life are unknown, aside from the fact that he lived in about 150 C.E. Patañjali is believed to have been an incarnation of Ananta, the mythical Serpent-King on whom Lord Viṣṇu takes his rest before embarking on a new creation cycle. Patañjali is said to have fallen into the arms of his mother as she was giving water to the sun in a gesture of worship. His name comes from *pata*—meaning both "serpent" and "fallen," and *añjali*, refering to the gesture his mother's hands made when touching in prayer. He is usually depicted in front of a thousand-headed snake, which drapes over his head like a suit of armor. He has four arms, in which he holds a conch shell, a disk, a mace, and a sword. In another depiction, he is half-man, half-snake, carrying the weight of the world on his hooded head or curled beneath Viṣṇu, for whom he serves as a kind of cushion or bed.

The author of the *Yoga Sūtras* is thought by many also to be the author—who also went by the name Patañjali— of various ancient texts on Āyurveda and Sanskrit grammar (such as the *Mahābhāshya*), though it is not clear whether the two authors are in fact the same. Those who believe that they are the same date the *Yoga Sūtras* to about the third century C.E. Those who believe that the works were written by two different people date the *Yoga Sūtras* to about the third century B.C.E. Patañjali's yoga as outlined in the *Yoga Sūtras* comprises what we refer to as classical yoga. The history of Patañjali is quite elusive, and Swāmi Satchidanada and others have suggested that Patañjali may have actually represented a group of people who together codified the practice of yoga in the *Yoga Sūtras*. See also Aṣṭāṅga Yoga, Yoga Sūtra.

प्रज्ञा
Prajñā

"Wisdom," "intuitive wisdom," "gnosis." Mahāyāna Buddhism holds that *prajñā*, or the "inner guru," is the highest form of wisdom, as it is the intuitive inner knowledge that comes from the essential self, a knowledge that exists beyond finite facts, logic, or information. See also Guru, Mahāyāna.

प्रकाश
Prakāśa

From the root *kāsh* ("to shine") and *pra* ("forth"). "Shining," "luminous," "radiant," "pure consciousness," "self-revelation." When one attains a state of pure consciousness, all is illuminated. This is one of the dual aspects of Paramśiva, the ultimate reality.

प्रकृति
Prakṛti

From the roots *kṛ* ("to make," "do") and *pra* ("forth"). The substance of the material world, primal or primordial nature. Also understood as "the Creatrix." All of *prakṛti* (nature/matter) is composed of three qualities or *guṇas,* which exist in combination in everything in the world. The three *guṇas* are: *rajas* ("active"), *tamas* ("passive"), and *sattva* ("balanced"). In the *Yoga Sūtras*, the material reality of *prakṛti* is composed of many levels: *pradhāna* ("foundation"), which is an eternal dimension; *sūkshma-parvan* ("subtle existence"); and *sthūla-parvan* ("physical existence"). In the Saṃkhya system—the influential Vedic philosophy of dualistic realism concerning the universe and creation—the basic principles of existence (*tattva*) are classified into *puruṣa* ("spirit") and *prakṛti* ("matter"). Because *prakṛti* is unconscious in nature, it is viewed as the polar opposite of *puruṣa,* the transcendental self. Yet, it is the interaction of these two eternal substances of spirit and matter that leads to creation. Finally, *mūla prakṛti* (मूलप्रकृति), derived from *mūla* ("root") and *prakṛti* ("creatrix"), means "the natural form or condition of things" and is another name for Śakti. See also GUṆA, PURUṢA, ŚAKTI.

प्रलय
Pralaya

From the verb root *lī* ("to dissolve") and *pra* ("away"). In the periodic dissolution and reabsorption of the universe, *pralaya* is the period of rest or repose, a phase of passivity in which the world lies dormant. This dormant period—like the fallow period before a harvest, when germination and cultivation occur—is just as significant as the period of action.

प्राण

Prāṇa

From the root *an* ("to breathe") and *pra* ("forth"), *prāṇa* means "breath," "vital air," "breath of life," "life-force," "vitality." This ancient Sanskrit term appeared first in the *Vedas.* Although it is commonly thought of as the external air we breathe through the nose and mouth, it also refers to the internal life-force energy in the individual, otherwise known as *ki* (in Japanese) or *chi* (in Chinese). The ancient sages first related the breath to the vital life-force energy. According to Vedic philosophy, there are five vital life forces in the body. These are: *prāṇa* (ascending air), *apāna* (descending air), *vyāna* (that which holds *prāṇa* and *apāna), samāna* (digestive breath; the energy that carries gross matter such as food to the *apāna* and brings subtle matter to the limbs of the body), and *udāna* (that which carries the energy of food and drink up or down through the body). The *Atharva-Veda* details seven types of *prāṇa*, seven types of *apāna*, and seven types of *vyāna.*

That the breath is so closely linked to the life-force energy is not surprising. Breath is the one thing that human beings cannot live without for any length of time. We can live for days without food, water, or shelter, but when we stop breathing, we stop living. As the *Haṭha Yoga Pradīpikā* states, "As long as there is breath in the body, there is life. When breath departs, so too does life. Therefore, regulate the breath." See also APĀNA, BANDHA, AṢṬĀṄGA YOGA (PRĀṆĀYĀMA).

प्राणायाम
Prāṇāyāma

From *prāṇa* ("breath") and *yama* ("regulation," "restraint," "control"). Literally, breath control, breath regulation, breath expansion/extension, and breath restraint. One of the Eight Limbs of Aṣṭāṅga Yoga, *prāṇāyāma* is practiced to deepen one's yoga, enhance the flow of life-force through the body, control the wandering mind, and achieve union with the Divine.

More than just breathing exercises, *prāṇāyāma* regulates the flow of breath to shift the flow of *prāṇa* in the energy channels of the *prāṇāyāma kośa*, or energy body. According to Swāmi Satyananda Saraswati, *prāṇāyāma* is actually the word *prāṇa* plus *ayama*, which means "extension" or "expansion." In this view, *prāṇāyāma* means "expansion of the dimension of *prāṇa.*" Dozens of forms of *prāṇāyāma* are practiced in yoga, often in conjunction with the use of the *bandhas* (energy locks) and *mudrās* (hand seals). Some of the most powerful and popular forms are:

Ujjāyi उज्जायी
"Victorious breath," a deep breathing through the nose in which this deep, loud breath is "victorious" over the noise of the chatter of the mind.

Kapālabhāti कपालभाती
"Skull-shining breath," a rapid, forceful diaphragmatic exhalation that energizes the brain and revitalizes the body.

Pūraka पूरक
Inhalation. Breath exercises that stimulate the system.

Kumbhaka कुम्भक
Retention. Distributes *prāṇa* through the body.

Recaka रेचक
Exhalation. Releases unhealthy air and toxins.

These breathing exercises calm the body and nervous system, restoring serenity. There are *prāṇāyāmas* for release of toxins from the bloodstream, revitalization of the internal organs, relaxation, and many other functions. See also APĀNA, AṢṬĀṄGA YOGA, BANDHA, PRĀṆA, RĀJA YOGA.

प्रसाद
Prasāda

From the root *sad* ("to sit") and the prefix *pra* ("grace," "favor"). This is a state of divine grace or mental acuity that is considered a gift from God. It can also be used to describe an offering to God, which then spreads among his devotees with God's blessings, tranquility, and serenity bestowed upon them. *Prasāda* is believed to purify all offerings.

पूजा
Pūjā

From the root *pūj* ("to worship," "honor," "serve,"

"collect," or "shine"), *pūjā* is a ritual offering or ceremony intended to honor or express appreciation or adoration for the Divine, while affirming or developing one's own inner Divinity. *Pūjā* rituals can be performed with an image (*mūrti*), icon, or other objects considered sacred. Traditionally, a devotee presents an offering to the Deity (*pūjā*), and is then granted an audience with or glimpse of the Deity (*darśana*); the devotee receives a sacred article of worship (*prasād*) with which to invoke the Deity. A *prasād* can be a mantra, *yantra,* or *mūrti. Pūjā* is an essential aspect of Tantra Yoga and Bhakti Yoga. See also BHAKTI YOGA, TANTRA.

पुरुष
Puruṣa

Also *purusha.* "Spirit," "individual soul," "spirit," "seer," "person," "indwelling form of God," "individual soul." *Puruṣa* has also been literally translated as "what lies in the citadel of the body." The word means "absolute spirit" or pure consciousness, independent of everything. It is eternal, changeless, and pure. *Puruṣa* ("spirit," "soul") is forever entwined in duality with *prakṛti* ("matter," "materiality"). *Puruṣa* can also refer to the "Supreme Being" or "God." Advaita Vedānta sees it as the "eternal witness," the "Supreme Self," or *paramātman.* See also Prakṛti.

राधा
Rādhā

Literally meaning "fortunate, successful," Rādhā is the name of Kṛiṣṇa's consort, the most adored of the Gopīs, or ethereal "milkmaids" of Vraja who were Kṛiṣṇa's childhood companions and devotees. The Gopīs are the embodiment of ecstatic, totally unconditional devotion to the Divine. See also Kṛiṣṇa.

राग
Rāga

A special form, structure or underlying framework of a melody in Classical Indian music, as in the melodies of the *Sāma Veda* verses and chants. *Rāga* melodies exist between two scales and modes, and each *rāga* has its own flavor (*rasa*) and mood (*bhāva*). They reflect the rhythms of nature, the changing of the seasons, the pulsing of the energy of the world. See also RASA.

राजयोग
Rāja Yoga

From *rāja*, which means "king" or "ruler," plus *yoga*, "union." One part of the Trimārga (Threefold Path of Yoga), the triumvirate of classical yoga that also includes Bhakti Yoga and Jñāna Yoga. Also known as classical yoga or the "yoga of kings," Rāja Yoga is codified in the systematic path to enlightenment

(Aṣṭāṅga Yoga) outlined in the *Yoga Sūtras*. While Bhakti Yoga is the yoga of devotion and Jñāna Yoga is that of knowledge, Rāja Yoga is considered the yoga of balance between devotion and knowledge. The Rāja *yogin* seeks to quiet the mind through meditation or mantra, freeing the mind from *saṃskāra* (the veil of illusion) so that it can embody purity and virtue, ultimately reaching a higher state of consciousness and allowing the individual to merge with the higher self. See also AṢṬĀṄGA YOGA, BHAKTI YOGA, JÑĀNA YOGA, PATAÑJALI, SAṂSKĀRA, YOGA SŪTRA.

राम
Rāma

From the verb root *ram*, meaning "pleasing" or "delightful." Also called the "Dark One" or the "Pleasing One," Rāma is the hero of the immensely popular Hindu epic the *Rāmāyaṇa* (The Story of Rāma), a twenty-four-thousand–verse epic written by the mystic and sage Valmiki in the third century B.C.E. Unlike the other great Sanskrit epic, the *Mahābhārata*, the *Rāmāyaṇa* appears to have been written by a single author. Both of these epics brought religious teachings to a popular audience through the adventures of an *avatār* (god who takes human form) who comes to earth to uphold and espouse moral and ethical virtues. The *Rāmāyaṇa* incorporates many ancient legends and draws on the *Vedas* to tell the story of Rāma, heir to the royal family of Ayodhyā. Rāma was forced into a fourteen-year exile in the forest by his stepmother—the second wife of his father, King Dasaratha—so that her own son, Bharat, could inherit the kingdom. During this time, Rāma's consort Sītā was kidnapped by Rāvana, an evil spirit who prevented people from freely practicing their religion. Rāvana, who was the King of Sri Lanka, was a devotee of the three main Hindu deities—Brahmā, Viṣṇu, and Śiva—and as such, he was invincible. But the people could no longer tolerate his oppression, so they went up to the heavens and asked the gods for help. The gods decided to send Viṣṇu down to earth, incarnated as Rāma, King Dasaratha's first son. His mission was to destroy the evil Rāvana. With the help of Hanuman, his extremely loyal monkey-headed general, Sītā is rescued, and Rāma defeats Rāvana and returns from exile to assume his rightful place as the heir to the throne, which he ruled for eleven thousand years. The *Rāmāyana* shows how

Rāma's selfless conduct, unconditional love, and ability to maintain strength and calm in the midst of adversity pave the way for good to triumph over evil. He demonstrates the moral virtues later codified by Patañjali in the *Yoga Sūtras* as the *Yamas* (Moral Discipline) and *Niyamas* (Self Restraint), the first and second limbs of Aṣṭāṅga Yoga. In the *Vedas*, Rāma is the Supreme Being or Godhead and is considered the total embodiment of righteousness (*dharma*). See also Aṣṭāṅga Yoga, Mahābhārata, Sītā .

रस

Rasa

From the verb root *ras* ("to feel," "be aware of"), *rasa* is used to mean "taste," "essence," "savor," "juice," and "nectar of delight." It also means "essence of things" or "delight in life." Indian aesthetics holds that there are eight types of *rasa*: *shṛṇgāra* (love between a couple; erotic love); *hāsya* (mirth); *karuṇa* (compassion or sorrow); *raudra* (anger); *vīra* (fortitude); *bhayānaka* (fear); *bībhatsa* (disgust); and *adbhūta* (wonder). Others believe there are two additional *rasas*, which are peace (*shānta*) and devotion (*bhakti*). *Rasa* also expresses the devotion and love between the Gopis and Kṛiṣṇa. See also KṚIṢṆA, RĀGA.

ऋषि
Ṛiṣi

Also *ṛishi.* From the verb root *dṛsh* ("to see"). The *ṛiṣi* is a seer or sage, someone who traditionally "heard" or "saw" the ancient Vedic hymns during deep meditation. To honor this lineage, each mantra has three demarcations, which are written in the scripture preceding the chants: *ṛiṣi* (the sage who first "saw" the mantra); *chandas* (the particular rhythm, meter, and flow of the chant); and *devata* (the Deity to whom the chant is addressed). To honor the *ṛiṣi*, the forehead is touched with the fingers of the right hand. To honor the *chandas* and the powers of speech (*vak*) that reside on the tongue, the mouth or lips are touched. To illuminate the *devata* and invoke the Deity, the heart is touched before offering the invocation; in this way, the soul of the *ṛiṣi* remains forever linked to the chant.

There are three classes of *ṛiṣis*: *brahmāṛiṣi*, born from the mind of Brahmā; *devaṛiṣi*, sages who were born of the Gods/Deities; and *rājaṛiṣi*, kings or royalty who became *ṛiṣis*. *Ṛiṣi* is also an honorific title given to great masters such as the sage Ramaṇa, who is called the Mahāṛiṣi, from *mahā* ("great") and *ṛiṣi* ("seer"). See also DRIṢTI.

साधन
Sādhana

"Practice" or "accomplishing." A particular spiritual discipline. Also a Tantric term for spiritual discipline, or the "path to Realization" that leads to *siddhi*, or perfection. The *Yoga Sūtras* contain a section on Aṣṭāṅga Yoga, the Eight-limbed Path, delineating the eight stages of practice (*sādhana*) that the *yogin* takes to attain awakening and union with the Divine. See also AṢṬĀṄGA YOGA, YOGA SŪTRA.

साधु
Sādhu

"Holy man," "saint." From the root *sādh* ("to go straight to the goal"). *Sādhus* often cover their bodies with ash, to symbolize having left the material world behind, or having "died" to their own desire. They often devote themselves completely to worship, renouncing worldly goods and trappings, sometimes sitting alone in mountain caves for years at a time without eating or speaking, sometimes wandering endlessly on pilgrimage and pursuing other devotional acts expressive of their surrender to a higher power.

Some sects of *sādhus,* including the Naga Babas and the Aghori *sādhus,* cover their bodies with ash from cremation grounds, wander naked, and have long, matted hair that reaches to the ground and beyond. They also follow austere practices such as those of yoga. In the subcontinent the wandering *sādhu* is a common sight. There are even some charlatans. The real *sādhus*, however, live completely independently, relying on nothing from the outside, even under extremely difficult circumstances. They are healthy, radiant, and clear, representing the ancient principles of yoga—independence, freedom, and living in harmony with nature. See also BHAKTI YOGA.

सद्लिंग
Sad-liṅga

The *sad-liṅga* are the six markers on the traditional path to understanding the *Vedas* (and, eventually, to enlightenment). The six *sad-liṅga* consist of: *upakrama* and *upasaṃhāra* ("beginning" and "ending"); *apūrvata* ("novelty"); *abhyāsa* ("repetition"); *phala* ("the fruits of one's labor"); *arthavāda* ("praise"); and *upapatti* ("understanding").

सहज
Sahaja

"True nature." The term means, literally, "born together" and suggests that empirical reality and transcendental reality are not mutually exclusive but in fact coexist. When they come together, we ourselves are realized, or "born" into our own true natures, our essential being.

शक्ति
Śakti

Also *shakti.* From *śak* ("to be able"). The "divine cosmic energy," "cosmic power," "force/potency/capacity of the universe." *Śakti* is the energy of the cosmos that maintains the universe and also makes it disintegrate. It is the name for the dynamic forces of the entire universe. Śakti is the spouse of Śiva, and the two create a cosmic dance of creation and destruction, birth and death. There can be no Śiva without Śakti, no Śakti without Śiva. Śakti is considered the feminine aspect of Śiva, the Divine Mother of creation. This energy is believed to lie dormant in each of us at the base of the spine, waiting to be awakened. See also Kuṇḍalinī Śakti, Śiva.

SANSKRIT FACTS & LEGENDS

The Sanskrit name for the Ganges—one of Seven Holy Rivers—means "she who moves swiftly."

Sanskrit is the language of three world religions: Hinduism, Jainism, and Buddhism. It is also the language of yoga, since all of the original texts on yoga and yoga philosophy were composed in it.

The *Gheranda-saṃhitā* ("Gheranda's Collection"), a classical manual of Haṭha Yoga, states that there are over 840,000 yoga poses or *āsanas*—one for each living thing.

Sanskrit isn't called "The Language of the Gods" for nothing. There are thousands of deities in the Hindu pantheon, and even their names have names. Lord Kṛiṣṇa for example, has 1,008 names, representing the multiplicity of forms the divine and its human and energetic manifestations can take.

SANSKRIT FACTS & LEGENDS

Early Buddhists and Jainists rejected the use of Sanskrit in their scriptures, wanting them to be accessible to common people in their own tongue. Instead, they used Middle Indo-Aryan.

According to Vyaas Houston, in the early 1980s, NASA announced that Sanskrit is the only unambiguous spoken language in the world, making it perfectly accessible to computer processing.

The Sanskrit alphabet is said to have its own Goddesses that protect it, expressed by the word *avipastha*—protector (*pa*) of animals (*avi*), or "established in those who protect the finite beings."

The Triple Blessing *Śānti, Śakti, Śambu* means "Peace, Power, Plenty."

समाधि
Samādhi

"Bringing together," "union," "contemplation," integration," "pure contemplation." The final limb of Aṣṭāṅga Yoga, sometimes called "bliss" or "enlightenment." *Samādhi* is the ultimate state of being, when the meditator merges with the object of meditation and the distinction between subject and object vanishes. In the *Yoga Sūtras*, *samādhi* is "meditation that illumines the object alone, as if the subject were devoid of its own identity." In the *Haṭha Yoga Pradīpikā*, *samādhi* is "that which conquers death and leads to bliss."

Samādhi is often translated as "ecstasy," meaning "to stand outside the ordinary self," but it has also been translated as "enstasy," meaning "to stand inside the Self." Both views are correct, as this is a state in which one is both fully embodied within the Self and fully detached from the Self, or ego. There are two main types of *samādhi*—one attained by deliberate effort such as meditation or concentration, and one attained spontaneously. The state of *samādhi* is sometimes interpreted as the beginning of moving into higher states of consciousness. Individuals experience samādhi in many different ways. *Samādhi* is synonymous with many Sanskrit words, such as *umānī* (negation of the cognitive mind), *manomanī* (fixedness of mind), *amarata* (immortality), *laya* (absorption, dissolution), *tattva* (thatness, truth, realness), *shūnyashūnya* (void yet not void, voidless void), *parampada* (supreme state), *amonoksa* (beyond cognitive mind), *niranjana* (without stain, pure), *jīvanmukti* (living liberation), *sahaja* (natural state), and *turya* (the fourth state; state beyond wakefulness). See also Aṣṭāṅga Yoga.

संसार
Saṃsāra

"All together," "flowing." From the verb root *samsṛi* ("to pass through"). "The world of flux, fluctuation and change," "existence," "carrying on." This term also suggests the "ocean of life and death" and the "wheel of time." It is considered the melding of Śiva's three powers, or *śaktis*: *iccha* (will); *jñāna* (knowledge); and *kriya* (action), which together create the diversity of the universe. *Saṃsāra* is a world opposite from the unchangeable, ultimate reality of nirvana, or *brahman*. See also Nirvāṇa, Śiva.

संस्कार
Saṃskāra

"Subliminal impressions," "veil of illusion." *Saṃskāra* also encompasses psychological imprints based on past behaviors, patterns, and experiences. The endless cycles of *saṃskāra* must be transcended by the individual in order to free the mind to achieve liberation. In the *Samādhi Pada*, or first chapter of the *Yoga Sūtras*, Patañjali writes: "When consciousness dwells in wisdom, a truth-bearing state of direct spiritual perception (*prajñā*) dawns. . . . This truth-bearing knowledge and wisdom is distinct from and beyond the knowledge gleaned from books, testimony, or inference. . . . A new life begins with this truth-bearing light. Previous impressions (*saṃskāra*) are left behind and new ones are prevented (Chapter 1, Verses 48–50). See also Rāja Yoga.

संयम
Saṃyama

Meaning, literally, "constraint," *saṃyama* is the "self-control" or "self-restraint" that develops when the last three limbs of the Eight-limbed Path of Aṣṭāṅga Yoga are integrated. These limbs are inward-directed practices—*dhāraṇa* (concentration), *dhyāna* (meditation), and *samādhi* (contentment)—that focus on an object of meditation. Their integration produces mastery over the mind and leads to bliss and union with the Divine. See also AṢṬĀṄGA YOGA, PATAÑJALI, RĀJA YOGA, YOGA SŪTRA.

संन्यासिन्
Sannyāsin

From the verb root *as* ("to throw") and the prefixes *ni* ("down") and *sam* ("completely"). A *sannyāsin* is one who has completely cast off or renounced worldy goods and things; a renunciate, hermit, or disciple of a particular guru or spiritual leader.

शान्ति
Śānti

Also *shānti*. From the verb root *śam* ("to be at peace"). "Peace," "contentment," "stillness." The eternal principle of calm and repose, which posits that while everything is known in the all-powerful silence, at the same time it is manifest in the Universe. Śanti is often chanted three times after prayers, to invoke peace. The peace invocation is also found in longer chants or hymns, such as the *Śanti Patha* of the *Puruṣa Suktham* in the *Rig Veda* (Invocation to Peace, The Song of Puruṣa, Chapter 10, Verse 90) in which peace is sought for all beings on earth. When combined with *Om*, this becomes a prayer for peace for all creation. This hymn was first "seen" by the *ṛiṣi* Narayana (another name for God, or *brahman*). The Deity it invokes is Puruṣa itself, "who alone adorns the unmanifest universe."

Śanti Patha

We seek that which gives us peace from sorrow--present and future.
We seek growth for the rite of sacrifice, and growth for the patron of the rite, the Yajamana.
May the Grace of the Gods be with us.
May well-being be granted to all mankind.
May plants and medicinal herbs flourish and grow.
May good come unto us from two-legged creatures, and may good come from four-legged creatures.
Om. Peace. Peace. Peace.

Mani Varadarajan, scholar and the translator of this chant, points out that the scope of this chant is vast, encompassing all living things—animals, plants and all beings on earth—reflecting the entire chain of being. Plants and herbs are praised, since they provide sustenance and healing. Ritual sacrifice was central to the *ṛiṣis,* who composed chants like this, as the Gods received their powers from the vibration of the mantras offered during the ritual of sacrifice. Sacred food (*havis*) was offered to the Gods during these rituals, and Agni, the Fire God, traveled between earth and heaven carrying the *havis* to the Gods. This is why the sages ask that their sacrifices flourish and that the patron of the sacrificial rites (Yajamana) also prosper. See also Agni.

सरस्वती
Sarasvatī

From *saras* ("flowing") and *vatī* ("having"), *sarasvatī* literally means "she of the stream" or "she who has flow." It is said to be derived from *sara* ("essence") and *swa* ("Self"). Sarasvatī was a river in ancient India and also the name of the Vedic Goddess who was the consort of Brahmā, the Creator of the Universe. He made her from his own body so that they could procreate and create the human race; she embodies Brahmā's creative force. Sarasvatī is considered the "Mother of the *Vedas*" and is beloved as the Hindu Goddess of the arts and sciences, and as the embodiment of nature. She governs learning, music, dance, painting, sculpture and writing, much like the Japanese Goddess Benten. Sarasvatī is a luminescent white Goddess who is said to radiate "more than the light of ten billion moons." She is depicted draped in a flowing white sari and is sitting on a beautiful blue and green peacock, or on the back of a white swan. She has four arms, representing her omnipresence in all worlds: the front two arms are said to symbolize her manifestation in the physical world, while the two in back symbolize her presence in the spiritual realm. Two hands hold a *vina*, the classical Indian instrument that resembles a lute. Another hand holds a prayer book made of palm leaves (to spread her knowledge for the benefit of all beings); and the last holds a *mala*, or circle of prayer beads, made of pearls (symbolizing the jewel of meditation and the path to enlightenment). According to myth, she bestowed the gift of writing upon the world so that her beautiful songs could be captured on the page. Sarasvatī is also worshipped as the Goddess of Wisdom and Eloquence, and those wishing to receive these gifts offer her their devotion. See also Brahmā.

शरीर
Śarīra

Also *sharīra*. From the root *śrī*, meaning "sheath" or "to waste away." *Śarīra* refers to the physical body, or that which perishes. In Advaita Vedānta, there are three elements to the physical body—the *sthūla-śarīra* (the "gross body"), *liṅga* or *sūksma-śarīra* (the "subtle body"), and *kārana-śarīra* (the "causal body").

The gross body is made up of the food sheath, or the physical body. The subtle body is made up of three sheaths: the sheath of breath, the mental sheath, and the sheath of consciousness/intellect. The causal body is the sheath of bliss.

शास्त्र
Śāstra

Also *shāstra*. From the verb root *śās* ("to teach" or "to rule"), this term refers to "scripture," "teaching," "doctrine," or "treatise." In addition to the Tantric doctrines, India has four kinds of scriptures. Primary scriptures are those that are heard (*śruti*) and passed down through the oral tradition; secondary scriptures include those that are remembered (*smṛiti*) as well as historical and mythological texts (*purâṇa*) and epics (*ithihāsa*).

The Yoga Śāstra is a text written by Dattātreya as a 334-line dialog between a sage (Dattātreya) and a seeker (Sāmkriti), in which concentration techniques (*sanketas*) are said to be a means of entering the void (*aūnya*). See also Sūnyatā.

सत्
Sat

"Being," "reality," "truth," "essence," "soul," "the best." The term *sat* is used to refer to "ultimate reality" (*brahman*). *Sat* is part of the sacred expression *Om Tat Sat* and is considered the self-conductor of everything. See also Om, Om Tat Sat, Tat.

सत्संग
Satsaṃga

Also *satsang*. "True company," "company of Truth." From *sat* ("truth") and *sangha* ("assembly"). Keeping company with sages, holy men, enlightened beings, and disciples. *Satsaṃga* also means a gathering of spiritual or enlightened beings, a community gathering, or, in more contemporary terms, "keeping good company."

सत्य
Satya

"Truth," "reality," "that which exists." *Sat* is the present participle of the verb root *as* ("to be"). *Satyagraha*, which is derived from this root, means "holding onto the truth." In India, Gandhi instituted a campaign of Satyagraha, or "Insistence on Truth," the most famous example of which was his model of nonviolent civil disobedience, in which he incorporated the principle of *ahimsā* (nonviolence) from the Eight Limbs of Yoga practice. See also Aṣṭāṅga Yoga.

सेवा
Sevā

Service. Offering one's time, energy, knowledge, experience, physical labor, money, teaching, or any kind of aid or service without expectation, acknowledgment, or reward. *Sevā* is one of the cornerstones of Karma Yoga (the yoga of selfless service) and Bhakti

Yoga (the yoga of devotion) in which selfless giving is a spiritual practice embodying the highest form of service.

In Radhakrishnan's version of the *Bhagavad Gītā* (Book 4, Verse 34), Kṛiṣṇa implores Arjuna to relinquish the ego and perform his duty with a sense of detachment and without regard for the fruits of his labor. The translator comments that "The goal is life-giving wisdom, which gives us freedom of action and liberation from the bondage of work." Kṛiṣṇa says: "Learn that by humble reverence, by inquiry, and by service."

The act of offering oneself to others breaks the bonds of ego and unifies us with the divine source. When we extend our hands in acts of compassion, the "giver" disappears, becoming instead a conduit for divine love. *Sevā* is an expression of nonattachment in action. Giving for giving's sake requires surrender and sacrifice, liberating and benefiting both giver and receiver in a transformational exchange. The spirit of giving is as important as the gift itself.

In the *Bhagavad Gītā* (Book 14, Verse 26), Kṛiṣṇa also invites Arjuna to worship him as a form of *sevā*. "He who serves me with unfailing devotion of love, rises above the three modes [sattvic, rajasic, tamasic]. He too is fit for becoming Brahman," he says. In the classic guru-disciple relationship, a student will also perform *sevā* by tending the teacher's household or performing other duties at the guru's request. As the student's ability progresses, her responsibilities increase. This is part of the learning process and preparation for deepening one's yoga. A *sevak* is one who performs *sevā*.

> I slept and dreamt
> That life was joy.
> I awoke and saw that
> Life was service.
> I acted and behold,
> Service was joy.
>
> —Rabindranath Tagore

सिद्धि
Siddhi

"Attainment," "realization." There are eight classic *siddhis*, or Tantric "powers." These paranormal potentialities in the human being are also known as *vibhuti*. Lord Śiva, the paradigmatic *yogin*, is said to have possessed eight attributes.

The Eight Tantric Powers

1. Aṇiman अणिमन्
The ability to shrink, to become "as small as an atom."

2. Mahiman महिमन्
The ability to expand.

3. Laghiman लघिमन्
The ability to levitate.

4. Prāpti प्राप्ति
The ability to extend, connect, bridge great distances.

5. Prākāmya प्राकाम्य
The ability to manifest will.

6. Vashitva वशित्व
Complete mastery over material elements.

7. Īshitṛtva ईशित्व
Lordship. Mastery over the subtle causes of the material world, when accomplished makes the *yogin* equal to The Creator.

8. Kāmāvasāyitva कामावसायित्व
Fulfillment of desires or the ability to suppress desire.

According to the *Yoga Sūtras* (Chapter 4, Verse 1) these *siddhis* are attained with yoga practice, meditation, *kriyā*, magic, mantras, *rasa* (elixirs), and *oṣadhi* (herbal potions). Someone who has attained the powers of the *siddhis*—an accomplished *yogin* or "perfected being"—is called a *siddha.*

सीता
Sītā

The literal meaning of the word *sītā* is "furrow." Sītā is the name of Rāma's beautiful wife, who is the heroine of the *Rāmāyana*. She is considered the ideal, perfect wife who stands for love, fidelity, and devotion. In the *Rāmāyana*, Rāma wishes to marry Sītā but, in typical princely fashion, he has to compete for her hand by bending Lord Śiva's bow in front of Sītā's father, King Janaka. While the other suitors are unable even to lift it, Rāma manages not only to bend the bow but actually to break it, and so he easily wins the beautiful Sīta's hand. Meanwhile, Rāma's stepmother is determined to have her son Bharat inherit the throne instead of Rāma, and she convinces the distraught

King Dasarath to send his oldest son into exile in the forest. Even though Rāma's brothers (including Bharat) are furious, Rāma consents to his stepmother's decree and takes his new bride into the forest. In the forest, Sītā explains the three sins: lying (false speech), being unfaithful in matrimony, and cruelty toward those who are not a threat. When Rāma is away, a sage comes to their hut begging for food. It is the evil Rāvana in disguise. He captures Sītā and kidnaps her to his kingdom in Sri Lanka. Eventually, she is rescued by the ultra-powerful monkey General Hanuman, who has bridged gaps between mountains with his legs and secured potent medicinal herbs to help his beloved master Rāma win the fight against Rāvana. (In fact, the yoga pose for the splits, *Hanumānāsana*, is named in the general's honor, celebrating his ability to stretch his legs across mountains.)

Finally, Rāma kills Rāvana, but because Sītā has been held in captivity in another man's castle, her chastity is questioned. When she is forced to sit in a fire as a test of her virtue, she emerges unscathed. Rāma and Sītā return to the kingdom of Ayodhyā to claim Rāma's rightful throne, but Sītā's chastity is still questioned by the general public. Although Rāma has no doubt of Sītā's loyalty and assures her of his faith in her, under public pressure, he asks Sītā to go through another test to prove her purity. Sītā, however. does not feel the need to undergo any more tests. Disheartened by the pleas of the public, she asks her mother, who is Mother Earth—Sītā is said to have been born from the Earth—to take her back in her arms if she has, in fact, been loyal to Rāma. The Earth opens up, and Sītā's mother takes her back into her natural abode. Sītā is also associated with the Goddess Lakṣmī. Though she is most often celebrated as the perfect wife, women around the world celebrate her loyalty to her husband and the strength she demonstrates in making this last decision on her own. See also RĀMA.

शिव
Śiva

Also Shiva. This term literally means "auspicious one." Śiva is variously referred to as "the Benign One," "Lord," and "Deity." The name also represents ultimate reality. As one of the three Gods of the Hindu Trinity, or *Trimūrti*, Śiva is commonly called "the Destroyer," but in actuality he represents not only the destructive force of the universe but also its restoration. He embodies these two seemingly paradoxical qualities and so represents the union of opposites. Through change and upheaval, Śiva destroys what is outworn, only to give birth to something better. He is therefore called both "Śiva the Destroyer, " and "Śiva the Regenerator." To many, he symbolizes the indelible link between the destructive and the ecstatic. As Swāmi Prabhavananda writes, "Śiva is often spoken of as "the Destroyer," but this is a misleading word, because the universe is never destroyed. Since it is subject to the eternal power of *brahman*, the universe is part of a beginningless and endless process, which alternates between the two phases of potentiality and expression."

Śiva has many manifestations. He is often depicted together with his wife, the Goddess Pārvatī and his son, the elephant-headed God Gaṇeśa. This Divine Family is said to represent the qualities of energy (Śiva), nature (Pārvatī), and wisdom (Gaṇeśa). In this context Śiva is often shown riding a bull (Nandin), symbol of sexual vitality.

Another image of Śiva is as the four-armed Nataraj, the "Lord of the Dance," dancing in a circle of fire. Here Śiva moves to the rhythms of the cosmic forces of life and death, creation and destruction, good and evil. His back right hand holds an hour-glass drum, representing the continual dance of the universe. His front right hand makes the "no fear" gesture, shielding from harm. His back left hand carries a purifying flame (*agni*), while the front left hand points downward to his raised left foot, which is balanced with poise and grace, reflecting release and everlasting bliss. The other foot is on the ground or stomping on the body of Apasmara, the dwarf demon of ignorance and suffering of those on earth.

Śiva is also revered by *sādhu* (holy men) as the archetypical *yogī*, and is most often portrayed in a yoga posture, draped in sacred beads (*rudrākśa)* and meditating in the Himalayan mountains. He is covered in purifying ash. His long, matted hair, through which the Ganges River is said to have dripped slowly to earth, contains the crescent moon, symbolizing the ability to control time. The jewel in his forehead represents the third eye, the center of inner wisdom. He is also portrayed with serpents wrapped around his neck and arms (symbolizing *kuṇḍalinī* energy), draped in tiger skin, grasping a trident (*trishul*), and beating a drum from which all of the sounds of the universe emanate. Nearby is the *liṅgam*, a symbol of Śiva's elemental form, rising from the *yoni* (symbol of Śakti) representing the creative principle of the universe. Śiva is considered the Father of Shamans and the God of Yoga.

Śiva's counterpart Śakti symbolizes the energy of the manifested Universe. The cosmic couple of Śiva/Śakti are interconnected and interdependent: one cannot exist without the other, and the energy of one informs the other. In fact, there is a saying, "Śiva is *Śava* without Śakti." (In Sanskrit, *śava* means "corpse.") Together, Śiva/Śakti are united as *brahman*, the Absolute Reality. In the Śaiva school of thought, Śiva is believed to represent creation (*sṛṣṭi*), maintenance (*sthiti*), dissolution (*saṁhāra*), obscuration (*tirodhāna*), and grace (*anugraha*). In Tantric philosophy, Śiva symbolizes pure consciousness while Śakti symbolizes power in the forms of *iccha* (will), *jñāna* (knowledge), and *kriya* (action). The practice of Tantra is geared toward uniting Śiva and Śakti as a means to *mokśa* (liberation). Another name for Śiva is Śambu, or "Horn of Plenty." See also Brahmā, Gaṇeśa, Kuṇḍalinī Śakti, Liṅgam, Pārvatī, Śakti, Ṣram, Trimūrti, Viṣṇu.

स्मृति
Smṛiti

From the verb root *smṛi* ("to remember"). Translated as "memory," "recollection," "that which is remembered," and "mindfulness." In the *Yoga Sūtras* (Chapter 1, Verse 20), Patañjali lists *smṛiti*, or mindfulness, as one of the five essential elements of the *yogin*'s successful journey to self-awareness. The others are: *śraddhā* (faith or trust), *vīrya* (vitality or energy), *samādhi* (contemplation/integration), and *prajñā* (wisdom/knowledge).

सोम
Soma

"Pressed juice." From the verb root *su*, "to press." One of the most sacred and mystic plants in the ancient world, said to yield the nectar of immortality. It is mentioned throughout the yogic scriptures including the *Rig Veda*, *Bhagavad Gītā*, and *Yoga Sūtras*. The ninth book of the ten *Rig Vedas* is actually dedicated to *soma* hymns. In fire ceremonies described in the *Rig Veda,* the *soma* plant was pressed between stones, mixed with milk, and filtered through sheepskin, and then consumed during the rituals. Considered a divine hallucinogen and energizer, *soma* produced a sense of superconsciousness and visions of the gods. According to Vedic hymns, "Soma" is also the name of the God who represents the juice of the *soma* plant.

Certain hymns extol Soma as the creator or father of all the gods. He is said to be divine and immortal and to bring immortality to gods and men. All the gods are said to drink *soma*, and Indra was an especially enthusiastic worshipper. Symbolizing *ānanda* (bliss), Soma is also referred to as the Moon God and lord of the waters. Chapter 9 of the *Bhagavad-Gītā* states: "Those who study the *Vedas* and drink the *soma* juice, seeking the heavenly planets, worship Me indirectly. They take birth on the planet of Indra, where they enjoy godly delights."

Contemporary studies in ethnobotany have tried to identify the *soma* plant. Harvard researcher Richard Evans Schultes, often referred to as the "father of ethnobotany," was one of the first modern-day explorers to investigate the use of sacred plants in indigenous American cultures. He and others such as Huston Smith have postulated a connection between the shamanic use of ayahuasca and *soma*. Modern theories hypothesize that visions induced by *soma*, ayahuasca, and other plant medicines provided the basis for the creation of Yoga and other spiritual traditions. Some of these theories also hypothesize an ancient link between ritualistic plant traditions in the Americas and Asia. See also Bhagavad Gītā, Ṛiṣi, Ṣram, Veda.

श्रम

Ṣram

Also *shram*. "Hard work," "effort," "exertion." *Ṣram* is the root of the word *āṣram,* or place of hard work, spiritual practice, and higher learning. It is also the root of the Sanskrit word *ṣamana*, meaning "ascetic," or "one who builds heat and practices austerities." *Ṣamana* is also an adjective meaning soothing, appeasing, conquering, calming. The shaman can be defined as one who lives within nature and perceives nature as the spiritual teacher/healer. The *ṛiṣis* who "saw" the practice of yoga under deep meditation were a type of shaman, since they resided in nature, receiving all nutrition and protection directly from natural sources. To this day, shamans in South America, Africa, Asia, and other parts of the world continue to receive great spiritual insight from the way their lives are immersed in nature. Contemporary yoga teachers are beginning to understand the link between yoga and its shamanic roots. Danny Paradise, for example, speaks of this connection extensively in his classes. See also Āśram, Śiva, Soma.

श्री

Ṣrī

Also *Sḥrī*. From the verb root *śri* ("to be aflame," "to diffuse light"). The term means "excellent," "venerable," "auspicious," "beautiful." It is also used to refer to success, prosperity, glory. A term of respect, Ṣrī (also spelled *Śrīh* or *Sri*) is often used as an honorific prefix to indicate the holiness of the person being addressed or discussed.

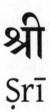

सुख
Sukha

"Ease," "peace," "inner joy." *Sukha* is a sense of lightness and joy, a sense of effortlessness and ease. It is one of the two qualities Patañjali delineates in the *Yoga Sūtras* that should be cultivated and nurtured in the practice of yoga *āsana*. (The other is *sthira* स्थिर, meaning "effort," "equanimity," "steadiness," and "alertness." Both are essential to the practice of yoga, comprising the yin and yang of Āsana Yoga.)

The literal meaning of *sukha* is "good space" and refers to the hub of a chariot wheel that is perfectly aligned and that therefore moves smoothly. The opposite of this quality is *duḥkha*, or suffering, which originally meant "bad axle space" that might cause a chariot to careen recklessly down a road. The *sukhaba bode,* or "abode of peace," is the quiet, joyful place within us where we can find inner sanctuary. See also Duḥkha.

शून्यता
Śūnyatā

From the root verb *śvī* ("to swell") and meaning "void," "nothingness," "emptiness," "nonexistence." In Theravada, this concept pertains to the individual. In Mādhyamika Buddhism, all is empty (*śūnya*), and it is this emptiness or formlessness that is the true nature of the universe. In Vajrayana, it is equated with the feminine principle—that which is unborn, vast, and boundless. The term is similar to the Japanese Buddhist expression *mu*, meaning "nothingness."

सूर्य
Sūrya

From *sū* ("to press out"), meaning "sun." Represents Divine Light. The Sun Salutation, or *sūrya namaskāra,* is from *sūrya,* meaning "sun" and *namaskāra*, from *na* ("not") plus *ma* ("mine") and *kara* ("to do")—a greeting given in the spirit of worship, essentially acknowledging "not of my doing, but of the Divine." The Sun Salutation is a sequence of yoga postures used to warm the body up and stimulate the flow of energy (*prāṇa*), building heat (*tapas*). The arms open out to embrace the sun and, at the same time, the heart opens and the *yoginī* joins her inner radiance with the light of the sun. In ancient times, *yogī* who practiced the Sun Salutation returned their life force to the Sun God with every breath.

सूत्र
Sūtra

From the verb root *si* ("to sew"), *sūtra* means "aphorism" or "thread." Mainly understood as a set of highly condensed or abbreviated aphorisms setting forth the concepts and precepts of a philosophical system. Each school of Hindu philosophy has a *sūtra* to provide a thread linking its tenets. Most *sūtras* were composed as mnemonic devices to stimulate memory, rather than as full explanations of a particular doctrine. As a result, ancient *sūtras* usually come with a commentary, called *bhāṣya*, to help explain their sometimes complex or obscured meanings. See also Patañjali, Yoga Sūtra.

स्वामिन्
Swāmin

Also *swāmi*. From the word *sva* ("to own"), *swāmin* refers to a "lord," "spiritual preceptor," "spiritual teacher," or "person from the upper castes." The term also literally means "learned Brahmin."

तन्त्र
Tantra

From the root *tan* ("do in detail") and *trā* ("protect"), Tantra refers to a "ritual," "rule," "scripture," or "religious treatise." Tantra is a religious science through which adepts seek liberation by awakening *śakti* (divine power) through Tantric rituals, or *pūjā*.

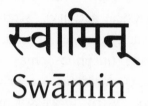

These rituals include the practice of mantras (sacred words), *yantras* (sacred/mystical diagrams), *upāsana* (meditation), *pūjā* (ceremonial worship, ritual), and *arcā* (image worship). The word *tantra* is said to derive, alternatively, from the Sanskrit roots for "body" (it focuses on physical activity), "stretch" (it extends individual capacity); "rope" (it binds the devotee to the Deity), "harp" (its philosophies are harmonious), "interiority" (its doctrines are private/protected), and "loom" and "warp" (it weaves together the cosmic principles of male and female that form the fabric of the universe). Tantric texts known as *tantras* (rather than *sūtras*) explain these practices, as well as detailing the *tattvas*—essential principles illuminating the "thatness" and "suchness" of things. The *tantras* reveal how everything in existence is woven together: all people, animals, and elements of nature are linked as part of the eternal One, while everything within the One interrelates. The *tantras* also explain the union of consciousness (*śiva*) and action or energy (*śakti*). According to the *tantras*, there should be spiritual consciousness behind all action and thought processes. Though modern interpretations link it mainly to the sacred nature of sex, *tantra* integrates spiritual awareness in *all* forms of action. See also PŪJĀ.

तत्
Tat

"That." This genderless pronoun expresses the Absolute, which cannot be described. A related word is *tathātā*, which means "suchness" or "things as they are," reflecting the essential, indescribable essence of things, an essence that transcends dualities. *Tat* is part of the sacred expression *Om Tat Sat*. See also OM, OM TAT SAT, SAT.

त्रिमार्ग
Trimārga

The Threefold Path of Yoga. The triumvirate of classical yoga, which comprises Bhakti Yoga, Jñāna Yoga, and Karma Yoga (see the respective entries for each).

त्रिमूर्ति
Trimūrti

From *tri* ("three") and *mūrti* ("aspects" or "faces"). This is the famous Hindu Trinity of Gods who represent the three facets of Isvara: Brahmā (from *bṛih*, "to expand"), the Evolver and Emanator; Viṣṇu (from *viś* "to enter," "pervade"), the Preserver and Sustainer; and Śiva (from *śiva*, which means "kindly" or "auspicious"), the Destroyer and Regenerator. See also BRAHMĀ, ŚIVA, VIṢṆU.

उपनिषद्
Upaniṣad

From the verb root *sad* ("to sit") and the prefixes *upa* ("near") and *ni* ("down"). Literally, "to sit down near," meaning "to place oneself close with devotion" or "sit at the feet" of a spiritual master or guru, whose words will impart wisdom. There are two basic types of *Upaniṣads*—Agamic (Tantric) and Vedic. In the latter, there are ten principal *Upaniṣads,* the final portion of the *Vedas* (also called Vedānta). The *Vedas* are the great oral teachings of the ancient Indian sages, which posit that humans can realize *brahman*, the Absolute Reality. The *Upaniṣads* are primarily concerned with the process of unveiling the true Self or *ātman* in order to distinguish reality from unreality. According to the *Upaniṣads*, individuals mistakenly identify themselves with their body, mind, and/or senses. Just as a shining moon appears to be a source of light but in fact only reflects the sun, one's true Self is reflected not by the body, mind, or senses but by a deeper, unchanging reality, which is the *ātman*, or soul. Through meditation and observation of moral conduct, one can ultimately realize that the true Self is identical to *brahman* or God. *Tat Tvam Asi*, "That Thou Art." This realization of Oneness, which ultimately leads to freedom, is actually not dependent on studying these revered scriptures. Rather, according to the *Upaniṣads* themselves, ultimate truth can be realized only through one's own experience. See also BRAHMAN.

वैराग्यमार्ग
Vairagya Mārga

Vairagya means "dispassion," "detachment," "non-attachment." *Mārga* means "path" or "way." *Vairagya mārga* is the path of detachment from worldly things, and of freedom from human desires. The seeker on this path gives up the pleasures of the flesh and the senses, renouncing the physical body to attain a higher spiritual manifestation in the body of a god.

वास्तु
Vāstu

From the verb *vas* ("to dwell," "to live"). *Vāstu* means "nature," "surroundings," or "environment." *Śastra* means "system" or "principles." Vāstu Śastra, or Vāstu, as it is commonly known today, is the ancient Indian art and science of designing and constructing structures to harmonize with nature, bringing peace, joy, prosperity, and balance to the building's inhabitants. The principals of Vāstu revolve around consideration of Earth, Space, Air, Fire, Water, gravity, magnetic fields, and the position of the planets when building. Important design principles include the shape of the land (the square and the rectangle are auspicious, while L-shaped or U-shaped structures or plots are considered unsuitable), the presence of bodies of water (north or east placement are especially good), and the avoidance of obstructions like trees or poles. Eight directions and their respective gods are central to Vāstu Śastra. These are: Esshan (direction: northeast), who gives wisdom; Indra/Angel King (direction: east), who gives prosperity and pleasure; Agni/Fire God (direction: southeast), who gives us charisma and the best things in life; Yama or Yamaha/God of Death (direction: south), who embodies the *dharma* and destroys evil; Nissan or Niruti (direction: southwest), who dispels fear and makes us victorious against our enemies; Varun/Rain God (direction: west), who rains down blessings, bringing wealth and joy of living; Vāyu/Wind God (direction: northwest), who gives us longevity, health, and endurance; and Kuber/Prosperity God (direction: north), who gives us prosperity and creature comforts.

वायु
Vāyu

"Air," "life," and "breath." Vāyu is also the Wind God—the vital force that links heaven and earth. While Agni represents Divine Will and Surya represents Divine Light, Vāyu represents Divine Energy. Vāyu inspires *prāṇa* and activates all the systems of the human body. Vāyu is traditionally called "Mātariśvan," or "he who extends himself in the Mother or the container." Here "Mother" could indicate the element of Ether or the energy of the Earth, which is referred to in the *Vedas* as "Mother." *Vāyu* is also one of the five gross elements (*mahābhūta*) that emerge from the subtle essences of the elements (*tanmātras*). These are: ether (*ākāsa*), which emerges from sound (*śabda*); air (*vāyu*), which emerges from touch (*sparśa*); fire (*tejas*), which emerges from color (*rūpa*); water (*ap*), which emerges from taste (*rasa*); and earth (*pṛthivī*), which emerges from smell (*gandha*).

वेद
Veda

From the root *vid* ("to know"), *veda* means "wisdom," "knowledge," "revealed scripture," "ritual lore." The *Vedas* are the most ancient and sacred of Hindu scriptures, or *śruti*, a word that originates in the root *śru*, "to hear," and means "direct from God" or "God reveals it." The four principal *Vedas* are believed to have been dictated by God in the fourth or fifth millennium B.C.E. and heard by highly evolved sages during deep meditation. The *Vedas* are thus said to be divine in origin, a reflection of Divine Truth itself—of that perfect knowledge which is God. They were subsequently passed down and recited by successive generations of priests in each of the specific areas of religious activity they address. They are the: *Rig Veda* (Hymns of Wisdom, which reveal the meaning of existence and of man's contribution to the world); *Yajur Veda* (Sacrificial Rites, giving most importance to the mechanical aspects of ceremonies); *Sāma Veda* (Liturgical Hymns, showing how music can elevate one's consciousness to the highest realm of Bliss and Supreme consciousness); and *Atharva Veda* (formulas to dispel evil, disease, etc.). The *Vedas* are comprised of four parts—*Saṃhitās, Brahmaṇas, Arāṇyakas*, and *Upaniṣads.*

The *Saṃhitās* are a collection of mantras that sing the praises of the many Hindu Gods and Goddesses while also rejecting pantheism and recognizing God as one Supreme Being. The many Gods are described as manifestations of the same Supreme Being, depicted in different ways. "That which exists is one. Sages call it by different names."

The *Brāhmanas* are concerned with everyday duties and rules of conduct. The *Brāhmanas* emphasize love, truth, kindness, and self-control and forbid theft, adultery, and murder. Emphasis is placed in serving the Supreme in all its forms—giving food to the hungry, medicine to the sick, and knowledge to the ignorant, etc. When performed selflessly, such actions or duties purify the heart.

The *Arāṇyakas* are concerned with the truths that are the basis for the forms of conduct described in the *Brāhmanas.* The *Arāṇyakas* are more concerned with a spiritual interpretation of the inner reality of one's actions than with the outward symbols of the actions themselves.

This deeper analysis of one's actions draws one closer to the last and most celebrated section, the

Upaniṣads. The *Upaniṣads* embody the essence of the *Vedas*, and are often called the "cream of the *Vedas.*" The *Upaniṣads* clearly define the prime Vedic doctrines of self-realization, meditation, karma, and reincarnation, and reveal the process through which one can achieve liberation through knowledge of the ultimate truth. Though orthodox Hindus consider the *Vedas* the highest authority, the teachings are not necessarily blindly accepted. The real study is to realize truth through one's own experience. See also Upaniṣad.

वेदान्त
Vedānta

End of the *Vedas.* This is another name for the *Upaniṣads.* It is also the name of the different schools of thought centered on its teachings concerning the nature of *brahman.* The major schools are Advaita Vedānta, which teaches absolute nondualism, in which it is believed that God (*Īśvara*), individual souls (*cit*), and matter (*acit*) are not separate and that everything is interconnected; Viśiṣṭādvaita, a qualified nondualism that holds that God, individuals, and matter are interrelated and that individuals and matter are dependent upon an independent God; and Dvaita Vedānta, which teaches dualism, expounding the belief that God, individuals, and matter are separate and distinct. See also ADVAITA, VEDA.

विन्यास
Vinyāsa

From *vi* ("in a special way") and *nyāsa* ("to place") and meaning, literally, "to place in a special way." *Vinyāsa* is often defined as "flow" and is a popular and relatively new form of Haṭha Yoga, born from the stream of yoga that originated with Śrī T. Krishnamacharya, which was then passed down to his students, who went on to develop their own immensely popular styles of yoga, including Iyengar Yoga, Viniyoga, and Aṣṭāṅga Yoga. Vinyāsa Yoga incorporates elements of each of those styles and other influences in a fluid, flowing movement that links one *āsana* to another like a dance. The concept of "flow" also pertains to the breath, as the flow is guided by the rhythm of the inhalation and exhalation, coordinating every movement with every breath. In this way, the body/mind/spirit are yoked in a dynamic interplay of breath and movement, stillness and motion. See also Yoga.

विष्णु
Viṣṇu

Also Vishṇu. The Supreme Lord, the all-pervading. One of the three deities of the Hindu Trinity of Gods, or *Trimūrti.* Viṣṇu represents the all-pervading reality and is known as "the Sustainer." He is the Deity who keeps the universe in perpetual existence. He is said to possess six divine qualities—knowledge, strength, divinity, power, virility, and splendor. When depicted, his skin is dark blue, and he has four arms. One holds a conch shell, one holds a discus. One holds a lotus, and one holds a mace. He rides on the back of Garuda, the great eagle. But this eagle is not just a majestic bird. It has been likened by Śrī Brahmananda to the "pulsation that arises from the movement of cosmic life," to which we must all listen attentively. Viṣṇu is said to incarnate on earth in times of evil or chaos to protect both gods and humans, and to reestablish order. Thus far, Viṣṇu is believed to have appeared in nine incarnations, the best known being Rāma and Kṛiṣṇa. See also BRAHMĀ, KṚIṢṆA, RĀMA, ŚIVA, TRIMŪRTI.

यन्त्र
Yantra

"To restrain," "to compel." *Yantra* are mystical symbols or diagrams designed to represent divine ideas or qualities and/or the *niruguna* (unmanifested) and *saguna* (manifested) aspects of the Divine. In meditation, they are used to direct psychic energy toward these aspects when the seer focuses his gaze on the particular pattern of the *yantra*. Eventually the diagram will be reproduced in the disciple's mind by the power of visualization alone. There are two types of *yantras*—those for protection and those for worship. In *yantras* for worship, there are specific diagrams for aiding in meditation, and those for calling forth divinities. In broad terms, Śrī Swāmi Satchidananda explains it this way, "A *yantra* is a physical expression of a mantra—a mantra being a Divine aspect in the form of sound vibration; a *yantra* in the form of a geometrical figure." He notes the expression from the Bible: "In the beginning, there was the Word, and the Word was with God, and the Word was God," adding that Sanskrit has a similar expression: "*Nāda, Bindu, Kalā,*" which means "the Sound, then the Dot, then the art of Rays," to express the manifestation of God. Since sound is invisible, the next smallest expression of the Divine is the dot, or *bindu*, which represents the core of the cosmos. But as it is too small to see, it expands out as *kalā,* the different aspects or rays of its manifestation. Those rays are expressed in the *yantra.*

Yantras differ from mandalas in that *yantras* are physical expressions of divine sound vibration, or mantras, whereas mandalas are separate entities representing holy abodes. Also, mandalas are based on circles, while *yantras* are typically based on square structures that contain circles, lotus petals, and triangles that lead to the center point, or *bindu*. See also BINDU, MANDALA, MANTRA, NĀDA YOGA.

योग
Yoga

"Divine union." From the root verb *yuj* ("yoke," "join," or "unite"), yoga is the science of spiritual, mental, and physical self-transformation. In rather broad brushstrokes, it is an ancient discipline that seeks union with the Divine—in other words, union between individual consciousness (*jīvātman*) and universal consciousness (*paramātman*). The root *yuj* originally meant "to hitch up" as in hitching a horse to a chariot. As scholar Barbara Stoler Miller has written, "yoga refers to both a process of discipline and its goal. It is the entire process that enables one to realize a state of absolute spiritual integration, which is freedom." Yoga balances the subtle energies in the body and the chakras, awakening the innate potential of the inner self, which is manifest at the gross and subtle levels. Yoga transforms the physical and spiritual life of the practitioner by releasing the physical, mental, energetic, emotional, and psychological blocks that limit potential; this release helps her evolve and grow. A sense of calm, balance, and ease follows. On the gross level, the practice of yoga has many concrete benefits, such as correcting physical ailments, reversing the aging process, providing strength and flexibility, purifying and detoxifying the system, toning muscles, regulating internal body functions, calming the nervous system, and curing a variety of ailments and illnesses.

The exact origins of yoga are uncertain, but these ancient practices and precepts predate written history. In the Indus Valley (now Pakistan), archeologists uncovered five-thousand-year-old carvings of adepts in yoga positions. This science was originally passed down orally from teacher to student, and was eventually codified by Patañjali in the *Yoga Sūtras* around two thousand years ago. Teachings on yoga were influenced by Buddhist, Jainist, Hindu, Saṃkhya, and Vedantic philosophy, and are also found in the *Bhagavad Gītā*, the *Upaniṣads*, and other sacred scriptures. Over the ages, different forms of yoga emerged to meld with particular philosophical and religious beliefs, like Bhakti Yoga, Haṭha Yoga, Jñāna Yoga, Kuṇḍalinī Yoga, Kriya Yoga, Karma Yoga, Laya Yoga, Mantra Yoga, Rāja Yoga, Tantra Yoga, and Yoga Chikitsa (Science of Yoga Therapy). Today, millions of people worldwide practice the many diversified yoga styles that stem from the ancient stream. Aṣṭāṅga Yoga,

Iyengar Yoga, and Viniyoga are often cited as the most influential of the "new" styles of yoga, but many other popular forms have emerged in recent years, including Anusara Yoga, Bikram Yoga, Integral Yoga, Kripalu Yoga, Satyananda Yoga, Siddha Yoga, Vinyasa Yoga, Yin Yoga, and more.

The concept of "yoga," or divine union, is found in cultural traditions throughout the world. For example, in the indigenous pre-Polynesian Hawaiian culture, the only law that existed was that "We are One." Similar to the yogic scriptures, this concept of oneness in the Hawaiian culture served as the basis of compassionate living since it was believed that all beings within the one are interrelated. Therefore anything done to one person is consequently done to the self as well. In Tibetan Buddhism one of the primary teachings is the interdependent nature of all phenomena.

The lack of understanding of the interrelatedness of all things and the true nature of the Self is considered one of the primary causes of all disease and suffering. Even modern theories of physics, such as the Theory of Everything (TOE), explain how all living things are linked by lines of energy as subatomic particles. Fritjof Capra, one of today's leading physicists, states: "The universe is fundamentally interconnected, interdependent and inseparable." See also Āsana, Aṣṭāṅga Yoga, Haṭha Yoga, Patañjali, Yoga Sūtra.

योगसूत्र
Yoga Sūtra

The treatise on yoga written in Sanskrit about two thousand years ago, reportedly by the ancient Indian philosopher Patañjali. A text composed of 195 aphorisms or *sūtra* (threads), stitching together the philosophical and practical system of yoga in which liberation (*mokśa*) is attained by stilling the fluctuations of the mind. The *Yoga Sūtras* begin:

> This is the teaching of yoga.
> Yoga is the cessation of the fluctuations of the mind.
> When fluctuations cease, the spirit stands in its true identity as
> Observer to the World.
> Otherwise, the observer identifies with the fluctuations of the mind.

The *Yoga Sūtras* are composed of four chapters, or

padas, that outline the progression of yoga practice. In the first chapter, the *Samādhi-Pāda* (Path of Ecstasy Chapter), Patañjali outlines the meaning and foundation of yoga. In part two, the *Sādhana-Pāda* (Path of Realization Chapter), he offers a description of the many ways yoga can be practiced. The third chapter, the *Vibhūti-Pāda* (Chapter on Powers), explains the *siddhis,* or powers that can arise from the practice of yoga; the fourth chapter, the *Kaivalya-Pāda* (Liberation Chapter), outlines the higher states of consciousness that can be attained through yoga.

The *Yoga Sūtras* also contain a section on Aṣṭāṅga Yoga, delineating the eight stages of practice (*sādhana*) the *yogin* passes through to attain awakening. Some scholars, however, believe that Patañjali did not write this section, but that it was added later to his original text by another writer. Debate about the author extends to uncertainty about the date when the *Yoga Sūtras* was written. Patañjali is thought by many to be the author of various ancient texts on Āyurveda and Sanskrit grammar that were written by someone also named Patañjali. Those who associate the author of the *Yoga Sūtras* with the grammarian Patañjali date the *Yoga Sūtras* as far back as the third century C.E. Those who believe that the two authors are different date the *Yoga Sūtras* to about the third century B.C.E.

To this day, the *Yoga Sūtras* remain one of the most widely studied texts on yoga and yoga philosophy worldwide. See also Aṣṭāṅga Yoga, Nirodha, Patañjali, Rāja Yoga.

योगिन् / योगी
Yogin / Yogī

"One who is joined or connected." Literally, "one possessed of yoga." A male yoga practitioner.

Book V of the *Bhagavad Gītā* reminds us that:

> Only that *yogī*
> Whose joy is inward,
> Inward his peace,
> And his vision inward
> Shall come to Brahman,
> And know Nirvana.

योगिनी

Yoginī

"One who is joined or connected." A female yoga practitioner. Interestingly, the word has also been defined as a "female demon" or "being endowed with power," or "woman representing a Goddess." We prefer the latter definitions, obviously.

योनि

Yoni

From *yauna* ("water"), *yoni* means "womb," "source," "vulva," "place of birth," "origin." The base of the *śiva liṅga* is a *yoni* with Brahmā, Śiva, and Viṣṇu inside it, emerging from it. In the Hindu trinity, Śiva is the destroyer, Brahmā the creator, and Viṣṇu the sustainer. The fact that the *yoni*, or female principle, contains these three incredibly powerful deities, symbolizes the root of *śakti* as the creator of everything—both Gods and humans alike. The *yoni* symbolizes receptivity, fertility, birth, Mother, the Universal Mother, Mother Earth, and the Goddess. See also Śiva.

CHANTS

Certain sacred Sanskrit words carry tremendous energy. Repeating the sounds at a certain rhythm, with proper pronunciation and deep concentration—a practice known as Mantra Yoga, or *japa*—releases this energy, giving sound a materializing value. The chants below are a few examples of the way that *ṛiṣis* selected words from ancient Sanskrit texts and arranged them so as to convey meaning and create tangible effects on our inner being. The soft vibrations still the mind, open the heart, and eventually balance our chakras, allowing for deeper yoga and meditation practice. Sound has been used in spiritual traditions and systems of psychotherapy throughout the world as a device for moving from the conscious mind toward the superconscious. These simple sounds have the power to connect man to the Divine and the ultimate unity in all things.

1. The following mantra is an invocation to peace. It is most often recited at the beginning of spiritual study or practice.

शान्ति मन्त्रः	*Śanti Mantra*	*Peace Hymn*
ॐ सहनाववतु । सह नौ भुनक्तु। सह वीर्यं करवावहै । तेजस्वि नावधीतमस्तु मा विद्विषावहै ॥ ॐ शांतिः शांतिः शांतिः ।	Om. Saha Nāvavatu. Saha Nau Bhunaktu. Saha Vīryam. Karavāvahai. Tejasvi NāvadhītamAstu Mā Vidviṣāvahai. Om. Śanti, Śanti, Śanti.	*Om*. May He protect us both (teacher and taught). May He look after us both to enjoy the fruits of our studies. May we work together with enthusiasm to find the true meaning of the sacred texts. May our knowledge and strength increase. May we never quarrel with one another. *Om*, Peace, peace, peace.

2. The *Gāyatrī Mantra* is one of the most sacred of the Vedic hymns, and is composed in 24-syllable meter. This mantra is also called the Sāvitrī, as it is addressed to the Sun God, giver of light. Especially powerful when chanted every morning, noon, and night, it is an ode to the power of *Om*, the sacred sound (*śabda*) that illuminates everything on earth. Chanting this mantra is said to give wisdom and aid in overcoming hardships and obstacles.

गायत्रीमन्त्र	*Gāyatrī Mantra*	*Mantra to Lord Gayatri*
ॐ भूर्भुवः स्वः तत्सवितुर्वरेण्यं । भर्गो देवस्य धीमहि धियो यो नः प्रचोदयात् ॥	Om. BhūrBhuvah. Svah Tat Savitur Vareṇyam. Bhargo Devasya Dhīmahi Dhiyo Yo nah. Prachodayāt.	Oh, Lord —Embodiment of vital spiritual energy, remover of suffering— you are effulgent like the sun. May you enlighten my intellect. May you give me wisdom.

3. The *Mahā-Mrityuṃjaya Mantra* has great curative powers. It protects against death and accidents of all kinds. This mantra bestows peace, wealth, prosperity, satisfaction, and immortality.

महा- मृत्युंजय मन्त्रः	*Mahā-* *Mrityuṃjaya* *Mantra*	*The Great Mantra* *for Immortality*
ॐ त्रयम्बकं यजामहे सुगन्धिं पुष्टिवर्धनम् । उर्वारुकमिव बन्धनात् मृत्युर्मु क्षीय मा मृतात् ॥	Om Tryambakaṃ Yajāmahe Sugandhiṃ Puṣṭi- vardhanam, Urvā-rukam-iva Bandhanāt Mṛtyor-muks. Īa mā-mṛtāt.	We worship Lord Śiva, the three-eyed Lord who is resplendent with fragrance and who nourishes all beings. May He liberate me from death for the sake of immortality, just as the ripe cucumber is severed from its bondage (off the creeper).

4. This is one of the most popular Vedic hymns celebrating the light of immortality and peace. Though appropriate for any occasion, it is often recited during Dīpāvalī, the Hindu Festival of Lights.

ॐ असतो मा	Om. Asato Mā	Lead me from
सद्गमय ।	SadGamaya	the unreal to
तमसो मा	Tamaso Mā	the real, from
ज्योतिर्गमय ।	JyotirGamaya	darkness to
मृत्योर्मा अमृतं	Mṛtyu r-Ma	light, from death
गमय ।	Amṛita. Gamaya	to immortality.
ॐ शांतिः शांतिः	Om. Śanti, Śanti,	*Om.* Peace,
शांतिः ।	Śanti.	peace, peace.

5. This mantra celebrates the Hindu trinity. It is a prayer to acknowledge the powers within and without, to create and preserve positive energy and destroy negativity.

गुरुर्ब्रह्मा	Gurur-Brahmā	Know the Guru
गुरुर्विष्णुः	Gurur-Viṣṇuh.	to be Brahmā
गुरुर्देवो महेश्वरः	GururDevo	(Creator).
गुरुः साक्षात्	Mahesh/varah.	He is Viṣṇu
परब्रह्म	Guruh. Sākshāt	(Preserver).
तस्मै श्रीगुरवे	Para Brahma.	He is also Śiva
नमः ।	Tasmai Shrī	(Destroyer).
	Gurave Namah.	Know him to
	(*Repeat twice*)	be Supreme
		Brahmā, and
		offer thy
		adoration unto
		him.

6. This popular mantra can be said at any occasion when one thinks of or wishes to invoke the Divine.

त्वमेव माता च पिता त्वमेव त्वमेव बंधुश्च सखा त्वमेव त्वमेव विद्या द्रविणं त्वमेव त्वमेव सर्वं मम देव देव ।	Tvameva Mātā Cha pita tvameva Tvameva Baṃdhush/Cha sakhā Tvameva. Tvameva Vidyā Draviṇam. Tvameva. Tvameva Sarvam. Mama Deva Deva.	You are my mother, my father. You are my family, my friends. You are my knowledge, my wealth. You are my everything.

7. The following mantra is a portion of a longer mantra traditionally chanted at the closing of an Aṣṭāṅga Yoga practice. It is a beautiful way to remind *yogīs* that the true purpose of practicing yoga is not for the self, but for the welfare of humanity. Through the science of yoga, individuals awaken peace, strength, and knowledge within, to ultimately share it with others.

लोकाः समस्थाः सुखिनो भवन्तु ।	Lokah Samasthāh Sukhino Bhavantu.	May all beings everywhere attain happiness and freedom.

8. This chant is sung in praise of divine female energy. Each goddess represents a different form of *śakti* (power, strength, and control), illuminated in the rich mythological tradition of the Hindu culture. Chanting their names together celebrates the mystical, deep powers of feminine energy.

दुर्गति नाशिनि दुर्गा जय जय । काल-विनाशिनि कालीजय जय । उमा रमा ब्रह्माणी जय जय । राधा-सीता- रुक्मिणी जय जय ।।	Durgā Nāshini Durgā Jaya Jaya Kal Vināṣani Kali jaya jaya Umā Rama Brāhmini Jaya Jaya Rādhā Sīta Rukamani Jaya Jaya	Glory to Durga, Kali, Uma, Rama, Brahmani, Radha, Sita, Rukmani—all Goddesses who vanquish darkness, ignorance, and unpleasant events. *Dur*: unpleasant *Gati*: events *Kal*: darkness/ ignorance *Vinaṣani*: destroyer/ vanquisher *Jaya Jaya*: Glory to (Note: Rama here refers not to Lord Rāma but to the Goddess Rama.)

9–12. The following four mantras are to specific gods and goddesses. When we pay our respect to the god(s), we acknowledge the Divine above as well as the divine qualities within ourselves. For example, when we chant the name of Sarasvatī, Goddess of Knowledge and the Arts, we acknowledge the Goddess for her creative energy, while also awakening our own inner source of creativity. While worshipping Śiva, Lord of Destruction, we acknowledge the powers above as well as within, to dissolve negativity and birth greater good.

ॐ गं गं गणपतये नमः ।	Om. Gam. Gam. Gaṇapataye Namah.	Invocation to Lord Gaṇeśa, the remover of obstacles, who guards the doorway to the enlightened realms. His blessings are essential for good beginnings.

या कुन्देन्दु
तुषारहार
धवला या शुभ्र
वस्त्रावृता । या
वीणा वर-दण्ड
मण्डितकरा या
श्वेत पद्मासना ।
या ब्रह्माच्युत-
शंकर-प्रभृतिभि
देवैः सदा
वन्दिता । सा मां
पातु सरस्वती
भगवती निःशेष
जाड्यापहा ॥

Yaa kundendu
tuṣārahāra
dhavalā
yā shubhra
vastrāvritā
yā veenā
varadanda
manditakarā
yā shveta
padmāsana
yā brahmā
chyuta śankara
prabhritibihi
devaih sadā
pujitā
sā mām pattu
saravatī
bhagavatī
nihshesha
jādyāpaha.

I pray for protection by Goddess Sarasvatī, who is white like jasmine flowers, brilliant like the moon, and sparkling like a necklace of dew, and who wears pure white clothes, whose hands are adorned by Veena and an auspicious staff, and who is seated on the throne of a white lotus, and before whom gods like Brahmā, Viṣṇu, and Mahesh always prostrate themselves, and who completely enlivens people's uninspired minds.

ॐ नमः शिवाय।	Om. Namah. Shivāya.	I bow down to Śiva, the Lord of Destruction. Śiva liberates through change and upheaval.
ॐ नमो भगवते वासुदेवाय।	Om. Namo Bhagavate Vasudevāya.	Invocation to Vasudeva, the one replete with Divine virtues, the granter of liberation.

13. The following mantra is often recited at the end of a spiritual practice or ceremony.

ॐ पूर्णमिदः
पूर्णमिदं पूर्णात्
पूर्णमुदच्यते ।
पूर्णस्य पूर्णमादाय
पूर्णमेवावशिष्यते ॥
ॐ शांतिः शांतिः
शांतिः ।

Om
Poornamadah
Poornamu-
dachyate
Poornaat
Poornamu-
dachyate
Poornasya
Om. Śanti,
Śanti, Śanti.

Om. That is
whole; this
is whole; the
whole becomes
manifest. From
the whole when
the whole is
negated, what
remains is again
the whole.
Om. Peace,
peace, peace!

BIBLIOGRAPHY

The following sources were gratefully consulted in the preparation of this book:

Andrews, Ted. *The Healer's Manual: A Beginner's Guide to Vibrational Therapies.* St. Paul, Minn.: Llewellyn, 1993.

Apte, V. S. *The Practical Sanskrit-English Dictionary.* Delhi: Motilal Banarasidass Publishers, 2004.

Chinmayanada, S. *Shri Krishnah Sharanam Mama.* Central Chinmaya Mission Trust, Bombay: Jay Graphics, 1991.

Coulson, Michael. *Teach Yourself Sanskrit: A Complete Course for Beginners.* Chicago: McGraw-Hill, 1992.

Farhi, Donna. *Bringing Yoga to Life: The Everyday Practice of Enlightened Living.* San Francisco: Harper San Francisco, 2003.

Feuerstein, Georg. *Tantra: The Path of Ecstasy.* Boston: Shambhala, 1998.

——. *The Yoga Tradition: Its History, Literature, Philosophy and Practice.* Prescott, Ariz.: Hohm Press, 1998.

——. *The Yoga-Sutra of Patañjali: A New Translation and Commentary.* Rochester, Vermont: Inner Traditions International, 1989.

Filliozat, P. *The Sanskrit Language: An Overview.* Varanasi, India: Indica Books, 2000.

Frawley, D. *Ayurveda and the Mind.* Twin Lakes, Wisc.: Lotus Press, 1996.

——. *From the River of Heaven.* Salt Lake City: Passage Press, 1990.

Gach, Gary. *The Complete Idiot's Guide to Buddhism.* Indianapolis: Alpha Books, 2002.

Gates, Rolf, and Katrina Kenison. *Meditations from the Mat: Daily Reflections on the Path of Yoga.* New York: Anchor Books, 2002.

Gopalacharya, Mahuli R. *The Heart of The Rig Veda.* New Delhi: Somaiya Publications, 1971.

Grimes, John. *A Concise Dictionary of Indian Philosophy: Sanskrit Terms Defined in English.* Albany, New York: State University of New York Press, 1996.

H. H. The Dalai Lama. *An Open Heart: Practicing Compassion in Everyday Life.* Edited by Nicholas Vreeland. Boston: Little, Brown, 2001.

Hearn, Lafcadio. *Strange Leaves from Strange Literature: Stories Reconstructed from the Anvari-Sohēīli, Baitāl, Pachísí, Mahabharata, Pantchatantra, Gulistan, Talmud, Kalewala, etc.* Boston: James R. Osgood and Company, 1884.

Integral Yoga Institute, Satchidananda Ashram. *Dictionary of Sanskrit Names.* Yogaville, Virginia: Integral Yoga Publications, 1989.

Isherwood, Christopher. *Vedanta for the Western World.* New York: Viking, 1960.

Iyengar, B. K. S. *Light on Prānāyāma: The Yogic Art of Breathing.* New York: Crossroad, 2003.

——. *Light on the Yoga Sūtras of Patañjali.* London: Thorsons/ Harper Collins, 1996.

——. *Light on Yoga.* New York: Schocken Books, 1979.

——. *The Tree of Yoga*. Boston: Shambhala, 2002.

Kent, Howard. *The Complete Illustrated Guide to Yoga: A Practical Approach to Achieving Optimum Health for Mind, Body, and Spirit.* New York: Element Books, 1999.

Kretschmer, H. *Sanskrit Bhagavad Gītā Grammar.* Vrindayan, India: Shri Krishna Balarama Mandir, 2001.

Kumar, N. *Basic Beliefs of Hinduism*. Khaknar, M.P., India: Manav Mandir Publications, 1986.

Lad. V., Dr. *Ayurveda: The Science of Self-Healing.* Delhi: Motilal Banarsidass Publishers, 1994.

McAfee, John. *Beyond the Siddhis: Supernatural Powers and The Sutras of Patañjali.* Woodland Park, Colorado: Woodland Publications, 2001.

Miller, Barbara Stoller. *Yoga: Discipline of Freedom: The Yoga Sūtras Attributed to Patañjali.* New York: Bantam, 1998.

Miller, Richard. *Mudra: Gateways to Self-Understanding.* Sebastopol, Calif.: Anahata Press, n. d.

Mukherjee, A. *Kundalini: The Arousal of the Inner Energy.* Rochester, Vermont: Destiny Books, 1986.

Pandeya, R. *Sanskrit Text for Human Excellence.* Delhi: Samskrta Kendram, 2001.

Paul, Russill. *Nada Yoga: The Ancient Science of Sound*, Roslyn, New York: The Relaxation Company, 1999.

Prahavananda, Swami, and Frederick Manchester, trans. *The Upanishads: Breath of the Eternal.* New York: New American Library, 1957.

Prahavananda, Swami, and Christopher Isherwood, trans. *Bhagavad-Gita: The Song of God.* Introduction by Aldous Huxley. London: Dent, Everyman's Library, 1975.

Radhakrishnan, S. *The Bhagavadgita*, New Delhi: Harper Collins, 1993.

Satyananda, Swami. *Moola Bandha: The Master Key.* Bihar, India: The Bihar School of Yoga, Nesma Books, 1978.

Schultes, Richard Evans, Albert Hoffman, and Christian Ratsch. *Plants of the Gods: Their Sacred, Healing and Hallucinogenic Powers.* Rochester, Vermont: Healing Arts Press, 2002.

Schultz, Larry. *Ashtanga Practice Manual.* San Francisco: It's Yoga Publications, n. d.

Simpson, Liz. *The Book of Chakra Healing.* New York: Sterling Publishing, 1999.

Sivananda, S. *Bhakti Yoga.* Rishikesh, India: Sivananda Yoga Vedanta Center, n. d.

Sjoman, Ṇe. *The Yoga Tradition of the Mysore Palace.* Delhi: Abhinav Publications, 1996.

Smith, Huston. *Cleansing the Doors of Perception: The Religious Significance of Entheogenic Plants and Chemicals.* Boulder, Colorado: Sentient Publications, 2003.

Spess, David. *Soma: The Divine Hallucinogen.* Rochester, Vermont: Park Street Press, 2000.

Svatmarama, Yogi. *Haṭha-Yoga-Pradīpikā*. Translated by Elsy Becherer. Commentary by Hans-Ulrich Rieker. London: Aquarian/Thorsons, 1992.

——. *Haṭha Yoga Pradīpikā*. Translated by Pancham Sinh. Allabadad, India: Bhuvaneswari Asrama, Bahadurganj, Indian Press, 1914.

Tagore, Rabindranath. *My School and An Eastern University: Essays*. Edited by Kizow Inazu and Kyoshi Yamaguchi. Tokyo: Tagore Memorial Association, 1959.

Toler, Celia. *The Yoga Year*. North Adams, Mass.: Storey Books, 2001.

Turlington, Christy. *Living Yoga: Creating a Life Practice*. New York: Hyperion. 2002.

Tyberg, Judith M. *The Language of the Gods: Sanskrit Keys to India's Wisdom*. Los Angeles: East-West Cultural Center, 1970.

White, Ganga. *White Lotus Foundation Training Manual*. Santa Barbara, Calif.: White Lotus Foundation, 1993.

Wood, Ernest. *Seven Schools of Yoga*. Wheaton, Ill.: Theosophical Publishing House, 1976.

Yogananda, P. *Autobiography of a Yogi*. Los Angeles: Self Realization Fellowship, 1998.

Online Resources

www.americansanskrit.com
Website of the American Sanskrit Institute, run by Sanskrit scholar and *yogī* Vyaas Houston, M.A.

www.ramanuja.org.
Great resource for those interested in learning more about Vedic and Upanishadic philosophy, chants, and more.

www.sanskrit.org
Website of the Sanskrit Religious Institute, offering chants and a wealth of information about Hindu religion and traditions.

www.sanskritstudies.org
A great reference for Sanskrit studies created by Sanskrit scholar and teacher Manorama, who offers classes and workshops in Sanskrit, chanting, and meditation nationwide.

www.samskrtam.org
Website of the Sanskrit Academy, promoting Sanskrit language and culture. Run by Sanskrit scholar Dr. Sarasvati Mohan.

www.yogajournal.com
Website of the print magazine. Great resource for those interested in any area of yoga.

www.yrec.org
Website of the Yoga Research and Education Center. Offers information on yoga history, philosophy, practice, Sanskrit, and much more. Run by prolific author and Sanskrit/yoga scholar Georg Feuerstein.

About the Authors

Leza Lowitz is a frequently published writer and yoga teacher who has been a student of Buddhism and yoga for over twenty years, since she was a teenager. She has a degree in English literature from U.C. Berkeley and a Masters in Creative Writing from San Francisco State. The coauthor of *Designing With Kanji*, she is also the author of three books of poetry, including the award-winning *Yoga Poems: Lines to Unfold By*, and a collection of short stories, *Green Tea to Go*, and the editor of many anthologies. Leza now lives in Tokyo, Japan, where she owns and directs the Sun and Moon yoga center.

Reema Datta has been exposed to yoga, Āyurveda, mantra, and Sanskrit since childhood. She has degrees in International Affairs from Vassar College and the London School of Economics (M.A.). Having worked for the U.N. and conducted research on women's empowerment in Varanasi, India, she appreciates this time in her life to explore the process of building empowerment from within. Reema has taught at It's Yoga in San Francisco, with Danny Paradise throughout Asia and Europe, and at Usha Yoga, a family-run studio in Maryland. Combining her interests of service and spirituality, she conducts retreats to Khaknar, a tribal village in north India where her grandfather runs a grassroots non-governmental organization.

BOOKS FROM STONE BRIDGE PRESS

Designing with Kanji: Japanese Character Motifs for Surface, Skin & Spirit
by Shogo Oketani and Leza Lowitz, 1-880656-79-5

Yoga Poems: Lines to Unfold By
by Leza Lowitz, ISBN 1-880656-45-0

Kanji Pict-o-Graphix: Over 1,000 Japanese Kanji and Kana Mnemonics
by Michael Rowley, ISBN 0-9628137-0-2

Japanese Yoga: The Way of Dynamic Meditation
by H. E. Davey, ISBN 1-880656-60-4

Living the Japanese Arts & Ways: 45 Paths to Meditation & Beauty
by H. E. Davey, ISBN 1-880656-71-X

Shinto Meditations for Revering the Earth
by Stuart D. B. Picken, ISBN 1-880656-66-3

Naikan: Gratitude, Grace, and the Japanese Art of Self-Reflection
by Gregg Krech, ISBN 1-880656-63-9

Available at booksellers worldwide and online